ENVIRON-MENTAL MEDICINE

OTHER KEATS BOOKS OF RELATED INTEREST

Are Your Dental Fillings Poisoning You? by Guy S. Fasciana, D.M.D.

Brain Allergies: The Psychonutrient Connection by William H. Philpott, M.D. and Dwight K. Kalita, Ph.D.

Candida: A Twentieth Century Disease by Shirley S. Lorenzani, Ph.D.

The Candida Albicans Yeast-Free Cookbook by Pat Connolly and Associates of the Price-Pottenger Nutrition Foundation

Diet and Disease by E. Cheraskin, M.D., D.M.D., W. M. Ringsdorf, Jr., D.M.D. and J. W. Clark, D.D.S.

The Do-It-Yourself Allergy Analysis Handbook by Kate Ludeman, Ph.D. and Louise Henderson with Henry S. Basayne

Good Food, Gluten Free by Hilda Cherry Hills

Good Food, Milk-Free, Grain-Free by Hilda Cherry Hills

Good Food to Fight Migraine by Hilda Cherry Hills

If This Is Tuesday, It Must Be Chicken by Natalie Golos and Frances Golos Golbitz

The Nutrition Desk Reference by Robert H. Garrison, Jr., M.A., R.Ph. and Elizabeth Somer, M.A.

The Poisons Around Us by Henry A. Schroeder, M.D.

A Practical, Participatory Course/Textbook

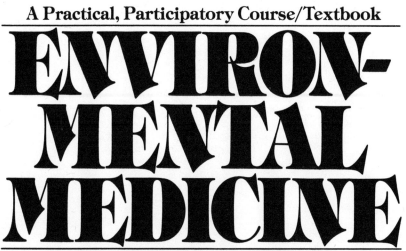

ENVIRON- MENTAL MEDICINE

— For Patients and Professionals
— For All Who Need to Know How to
Diagnose and Manage Allergies

**Natalie Golos
James F. O'Shea, M.D.
and Francis J. Waickman, M.D.
with Frances Golos Golbitz**

Research Assistant: Maryann Lazer

Keats Publishing, Inc., 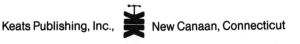 New Canaan, Connecticut

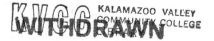

ENVIRONMENTAL MEDICINE. A Practical Participatory Course Textbook by Natalie Golos, James A. O'Shea and Francis J. Waickman, M.D., with Frances Golos Golbitz

Copyright © 1987 by Natalie Golos

Library of Congress Cataloging-in-Publication Data

Environmental medicine.

  Bibliography: p.
  Includes index.
    1. Environmentally induced diseases. I. Golos,
Natalie. [DNLM: 1. Allergens. 2. Environmental
Health—education. 3. Environmental Pollutants—
adverse effects. 4. Patient Education—methods.
WA 18 E615]
RB152.E575 1986   616.9′8   87-4082
ISBN 0-87983-425-0 (pbk.)

Printed in the United States of America

Keats Publishing, Inc.
27 Pine Street, New Canaan, Connecticut 06840

DEDICATION

To Lawrence Dickey, M.D., for his years of service as
Continuing Medical Educational Director of the
Society for Clinical Ecology program for physicians
and their staffs.

and

To the American Academy of Environmental Medicine
and its physicians for the courage to change
medical practice to meet the needs of the twentieth
century.

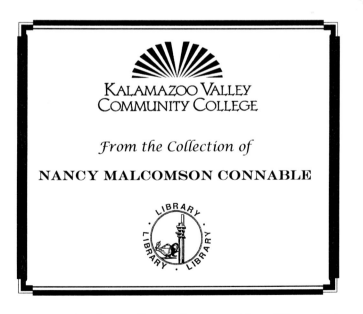

A C K N O W L E D G M E N T S

Very special thanks to Maryann Lazer for research and development of the bibliography and the list of cross references, for her clinical application trials, and critique of the teaching material.

Our special gratitude to Eileen Buckholtz, R.N., Jane Roller, Vera Rea, Glyn Nelson, Susan Meggs, Sheri Rechsteiner, Renée Lazer, Marie Waickman, Doris Cooper, R.N., Drs. James Brodsky, James Cox, William Crook, Lawrence Dickey, Alan Levin, Malcolm Maley, William Meggs, Theron Randolph, and William Rea.

Grateful acknowledgment is made to Dr. William Rea for permission to reprint his papers on alcohol, formaldehyde, phenol and the use of tri alkali salts.

NOTE: The word "he" is used in the book as shorthand for "he" and "she." It is not meant to imply gender discrimination, male superiority, or the authors' laziness.

Contents

Foreword, xi
Preface, xii

PART I: The Course, 1

INTRODUCTION, 3
Preview, 3   Objectives, 3   Some Authoritative Views, 3   A Typical Case
Study, 5   Basic Books, 7

ASSIGNMENT FOR CLASS ONE, 10

CLASS ONE, 11
Preview, 11   Objectives of the Course, 11   Objectives of Each Class, 13
Course Design, 13   Assignments, 14   Importance of Attitude, 15   Importance
of Education, 15   Some Brief Definitions, 16   Precautions, 18

ASSIGNMENT FOR CLASS TWO, 20

CLASS TWO, 21
Preview, 21   Objectives, 21   Something Is Wrong!, 22   Allergists and Clinical
Ecologists, 23   Symptoms of Ecologic Illness, 23   Food Sensitivity, 24
Variables to Consider, 26   Beginning Rotation, 27   Yeasts, 27   Sample Diet, 28
Saving Money, 31   Cosmetics, 31   Cleaning, 32   Entertaining, 33   Food, 33
Gasoline, 35   Packaging, 36

ASSIGNMENT FOR CLASS THREE, 38

CLASS THREE, 40
Preview, 40   Objectives, 40   The Chemical Questionnaire, 41   Interpreting
the Questionnaire, 48   Cleaning, 49   Products to Avoid, 49   New Products, 50
How to Use Bon Ami Bar Soap, 51   How to Use Rugged Red, 53
How to Use Organic Green, 53   Neolife Dishwashing Detergent, 54
Cautionary Notes, 54

ASSIGNMENT FOR CLASS FOUR, 56

CLASS FOUR, 57
Preview, 57   Objectives, 57   The Immune System, 58   Doing Your Own
Testing, 64   Your Temperature and Pulse, 65   Physical Changes, 65
Time Between Tests, 66   Food Testing, 66   Food Additive Testing, 68
Simple Tests for Airborne Chemicals, 69

ASSIGNMENT FOR CLASS FIVE, 72

CLASS FIVE, 74
Preview, 74   Objectives, 74   Detecting the Problems, 75   The Toxic-Free
Life, 75   Breathing, 75   Coping with Unavoidable Daily Exposures, 76

Before You Go Out, 77   While You Are Out, 77   When You Return Home, 78
Yeast Revisited, 79

ASSIGNMENT FOR CLASS SIX, 82

CLASS SIX, 83
Preview, 83   Objectives, 83   Type 1/Type 2 Reading, 84   Rebuilding
Adaptation, 84   Family Cooperation, 91   Do's and Don'ts for the Patient, 92
Do's and Don'ts for the Family, 93   Where to Take a Firm Stand, 94
The Importance of Support Groups, 94   A Final Word, 97

PART II: How to Teach Environmental Medicine, 99

INTRODUCTION TO COUNSELING THE PATIENT, 101
Successful Teaching, 101   Motivation, 102   Motivation of the Teacher, 103
Importance of the Counselor's Role, 103   Goals, 104   Tips for the New
Teacher, 106   Do's and Don'ts for the Group Counselor, 107

PART III: Lesson Plans, 109

PRECLASS INSTRUCTIONS, 111
LESSON PLAN FOR CLASS ONE, 113
LESSON PLAN FOR CLASS TWO, 115
LESSON PLAN FOR CLASS THREE, 123
LESSON PLAN FOR CLASS FOUR, 126
LESSON PLAN FOR CLASS FIVE, 130
LESSON PLAN FOR CLASS SIX, 139
A FINAL WORD TO THE COUNSELOR, 142
LIST OF CROSS-REFERENCES, 143
BIBLIOGRAPHY, 172
Appendix A: Formaldehyde Fact Sheet, 176
Appendix B: Alcohol Fact Sheet, 179
Appendix C: Phenol Fact Sheet, 181
Appendix D: Tri Alkali Salts Fact Sheet, 183
Appendix E: Use of Milk of Magnesia, 186
Appendix F: HEAL Membership Application, 187

Foreword

After being asked to write a foreword for this book, I made a pleasant discovery. I was surprised and honored to find it was being dedicated to me for my work as Continuing Medical Educational Director of the Society for Clinical Ecology and to others who had participated over the years in teaching the concepts and techniques of clinical ecology to physicians, nurses, and technicians.

For management to be successful, the patient must play an active role in his own care. To aid in this work, individuals have formed support groups such as HEAL, a national organization with local chapters.

Over the years, more than fifty good books have been published to help with patient education. The present work is an effort to organize a teaching program based on some of this literature.

There is an outline for six one- to two-hour class sessions, with reading assignments from six reference volumes. It can be profitably used for patient self-education. It is designed also for use as an instructional course to be conducted by experienced counselors. This latter approach could be especially effective as a special project for local support groups.

This educational endeavor is quite comprehensive in covering the non-invasive concepts and techniques of clinical ecology. These techniques are applicable in any medical practice where the physician is involved in patient care.

The royalties from publication are designated to help finance the preservation of Dr. Theron Randolph's library.

Lawrence D. Dickey, M.D.

Preface

This book is a teaching guide for the field of environmental medicine (the discipline of clinical ecology). We have written it with several objectives in mind.

1) to capture the attention of healthy people who wish to learn how to prevent chronic illness;

2) to alert chronically ill people to the fact that there is a field of medical practice that can provide help where there was none before;

3) to help former environmentally ill patients keep up with new trends in order to prevent their backsliding into careless habits dangerous to their health;

4) to teach patients who have completed their testing but are still under treatment;

5) to counsel current patients enrolled by their doctors in a class conducted by his trained professional staff.

Every book on environmental illness includes the first four objectives. But there is little agreement on how best to achieve these objectives and even less on their order of importance. For this reason, this material is presented as a textbook which teaches the reader how to study all the available literature, how to apply it to themselves now and what will be applicable in the future.

The fifth objective is a totally new concept because it was written primarily for use in a classroom situation. As a textbook, it employs good teaching methods with good motivation, lesson plans, interpretation of charts, etc.

Originally, it was to be presented as two books, one for patients to use as a textbook on environmental medicine and one for the doctors' staff as a guide on how to teach the course. The concept was changed to make both parts available to the patient so that it can be used after the class as a tool for continuing education and so that readers can be their own teacher. Both parts are available also to accommodate readers who wish to educate themselves with telephone supervision of a physician's staff when necessary.

The doctor's staff will be able to guide patients during the course of the class to show them how to teach themselves. That is how environmental medicine differs from most medical specialties; the main goal subsequently is to wean the patient away from the doctor and to teach the patient to be more self-sufficient.

CAUTION!

This book is not intended to replace your doctor. In fact, it was written primarily to be a teaching tool for the staff of the physician who practices clinical ecology.

If there is no class conducted close enough for you to attend, and if you have never been to a clinical ecologist, contact the American Academy of Environmental Medicine to find the nearest one to you, so that you can take the course yourself under his guidance.

AMERICAN ACADEMY OF ENVIRONMENTAL MEDICINE
P.O. BOX 16106
DENVER, COLORADO 80216

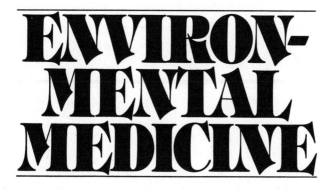

PART I

The Course

Introduction

PREVIEW

Environmental illness is not an exotic disease. Most of us currently suffer from it, but many have not identified it as the cause of their suffering. To the sufferers, environmental medicine is of utmost importance. Those of us who are proud of "being well" are advised to educate ourselves about preventing environmental illness. The first section of this book, then, is devoted to raising the consciousness of the reader to the world of allergies and the physical, behavioral, and psychological toll they can effect. This introduction will discuss *how* to raise our consciousness by using this book as an instructional tool and continuing reference. Its goal is the good health of the reader. The reader is the patient and partner of the professional health specialist in the attainment of this goal.

OBJECTIVES OF THE INTRODUCTION

After studying the course introduction, you should:

1 Know the purpose of this course as a guide to good health.

2 Understand the importance of education in the field of environmental medicine.

3 Understand the role of the clinical ecologist, *vis a vis* the traditional medical doctor.

4 Know the initial precautions to take to avoid environmental illness.

5 Be able to use bibliographic references in the field of environmental medicine for your personal wellbeing, as well as that of family members.

Some Authoritative Views

What is environmental illness?

What is environmental medicine?

Perhaps the best way to give you an initial understanding of these topics is to quote a few authors whose works will be introduced later in this book.

In the preface to her book, *Allergies and the Hyperactive Child*, Dr. Doris J. Rapp begins by saying:

When we think about allergies, we usually conjure up an an image of sneezing, runny noses; itchy, teary eyes; wheezing and coughing; or rashes. Less commonly recognized symptoms include muscle aches, headaches, dizziness, fatigue.

What about children and adults who are often depressed and irritable, overly active, belligerent, or poor learners? You may know, or may be the parent of, a child who is hard to discipline, continuously disruptive, and barely accepted by peers and siblings because of hostile and erratic behavior. Some allergists and pediatricians believe these symptoms can also be due to allergies.

As a pediatric allergist, I began to notice that some children treated for allergies appear to have fewer behavior and activity problems. Patients treated for hay fever, asthma, or eczema improve dramatically in disposition. Their activity levels sometimes seemed more normal and their schoolwork improved. Some parents also noted that their children's chronic muscle aches, leg aches and headaches subsided.

In the preface to *Coping with Your Allergies* by Natalie Golos and Frances Golos Golbitz, Natalie Golos introduced environmental illness (and allergies) in this way:

The pesticide massacre in Bhopal, India! Love Canal! Toxic waste sites! These disasters capture your attention, but do you feel you are personally affected?... the truth is, we are all victims of chemical pollution in varying degrees. Unfortunately, those who recognize it are few in number. And that is why this book has been written—to draw attention to the long-range perils and the chronic illness that may threaten you from long-term low-grade exposure to chemicals in your everyday environment.

...it happened [to me]—a kitchen stove gas leak, a leaky oil burner, and a direct exposure to insecticide. I had been so physically strong that it took all three direct exposures to reduce me from robust good health to life-threatening illness. But I was one of the fortunate ones. I found my way to a clinical ecologist who helped me find the long road back. Also known as environmental medicine, clinical ecology is the study of an individual's reaction to his environment.

Perhaps the most definitive explanation of environmental illness is printed on the jacket of *An Alternative Approach to Allergies*, by Theron G. Randolph, M.D. and Ralph W. Moss, Ph.D.:

At least half of the men and women in the United States suffer from allergies, and millions more are afflicted with continuing, chronic illnesses.... From his 45 years of practice as an allergist, Dr. Theron G. Randolph has discovered that allergies are similar to addictions in their early states; people can become addicted to common foods such as corn, wheat and beef, as well as to coffee, tea and tobacco. For those who are susceptible, everyday chemicals (gas from the kitchen range, supermarket food additives) can be a cause of mental and physical disease.

A Typical Case Study

In the books included in this course are hundreds of cases of environmentally ill patients, many of whose illnesses are life threatening. However, to indicate the nature of this illness and to show how widespread it is, we shall cite a case of an average person who has the problem, does not know it and is offended by the mere suggestion that he has environmental illness. We shall quote him directly from his introduction to *An Alternative Approach to Allergies* which he coauthored with Dr. Randolph. Ralph W. Moss, Ph.D. states:

I did not go to Randolph's Chicago office as a patient but as the coauthor of this book. On my first day as the Randolphs' house guest I looked around the breakfast table for my morning coffee. I was informed, politely, that the Randolphs never drank coffee. This made me uneasy, for I had had at least one cup of coffee almost every day of my life for the previous twenty years. At that time in fact, I was following one of the weight-reduction diets which calls for a cup of coffee or tea with every meal. Finally, seeing my distress, Tudy Randolph dug in the back of her cupboard and brought out an old jar of decaffeinated coffee which she kept for just such occasions.

In casual conversation later that day, Randolph dropped a reference to my "coffee addiction." I was surprised and a bit hurt that he would group me in the same category as the patients we were to write about. To prove that he was wrong, I vowed silently not to touch coffee for the duration of my stay in Chicago.

This resolution lasted three days. By the third day, I was literally falling off my seat in exhaustion—a reaction which the reader will better understand after reading this book. In the middle of an important meeting in Randolph's office, I had to excuse myself. I walked briskly to downtown Chicago, valiantly bypassing dozens of restaurants where coffee pots steamed on their burners or shoppers lifted their cups enticingly. I needed a fix! Just when I thought I had the problem licked, I walked past a French-style café in the Water Tower shopping complex. The odor of fresh ground coffee wafted out at me, and it was not long before I was seated before a big, hot mug of delicious java.

Before I could finish the cup, however, a headache, like a point of pressure in either temple, had started up. In addition, my heart began to flutter like a butterfly. I was astounded, for these were my two major medical problems. Frequent headaches, especially upon rising, had been with me since—well, since I had started drinking coffee, twenty years before. The worrisome, butterfly-like palpitations had begun more recently, a few weeks earlier. I later realized that the palpitations had begun just after I had doubled my coffee intake on the quick-weight-loss diet.

Aspirin was what I always resorted to when I got a headache, but this time I was out of luck. The Randolphs do not own any aspirin or any other pain killers. In fact, I could find no drugs whatsoever. A doctor without drugs seemed like a crime against nature! Never had I felt such pain as this "cold turkey" treatment for my coffee headache. I could neither lie down nor get up, stay in the darkness nor stand the light; even the tiny nightlight seared my eyeballs. I had simply never had to go the whole distance with my headache before, and I had not been aware of just how bad this problem had become. I had always been able to turn it off with those handy little white tablets.

After that experience, I stayed away from coffee for several months—more or less. On the few occasions on which I tried to drink it again, the headache and palpitations returned. After six months or so, I was able to resume drinking decaffeinated coffee, but only once every four days, according to the principles of the Rotary Diversified Diet, which will be explained later.

Basic Books

There is so much literature on environmental medicine (clinical ecology) that even physicians, when they are first investigating the field, find it difficult to know where to begin. This course should overcome that difficulty by helping you educate *yourself* and by showing you where to go to find the answers to your questions about restoring and maintaining your health. The authors have kept in mind that you are not going to remember everything that is taught to you in this course. Our main goal, then, is to show you how and where to go to get information when you need it.

The course is organized around the patient books of the pioneer authors in clinical ecology, which we believe is the best way to present the basics of the field. It also includes two books that add a dimension to the field and introduce some new concepts. There are other relevant books that would be helpful during the six sessions of this course. At the end of the course you will find a bibliography of other important books on environmental medicine. As you read the books, you will find a great deal of repetition and agreement. You will also note some disagreement and controversy. This, too, is healthy because it is thought provoking. If you are in doubt as to whether or not a particular viewpoint applies to you, request a consultation with your physician to discuss the matter.

You may find copies of the books you need for this course in your library. When you complete your reading assignments or cross-reference topics in other books, you may consider which of these books you will want for your personal library. It may be helpful, then, to review some criteria for selecting books that you will want to keep. In deciding which books you will borrow and which ones you will wish to buy, keep the following in mind:

BOOKS FOR REFERENCE   You will want to own books that contain practical, useful information to serve as guides to everyday living with allergies.

BOOKS FOR PHILOSOPHY AND SCOPE   You will want books that explain the theory, history and evolution of clinical ecology and that include case studies that demonstrate the value of this type of medical practice. Such books will be invaluable tools in helping you explain your health problems and needs, especially when you talk with friends, family, tradespeople, and uninformed medical practitioners.

SOURCE BOOKS   You will want books to guide you to sources of products that you will need but are difficult to find.

ASSIGNMENT FOR CLASS ONE

I. For the first session, read and be prepared to discuss Class One (the objectives, design and importance of the course and the suggested precautions you can take).

II. List *your* precautions by priority.

III. Complete the assigned readings in the books listed in Class One. Return to the particular reading to find the answers to the questions. Answer all questions before browsing in the books for other points of interest to you.

   A. *If This Is Tuesday, It Must Be Chicken*

      1. Philosophy and Scope

   Read: Foreword and Preface.

      2. Changing Your Eating Habits

   Read: Chapters 1 and 2.

      a. Name three sweeteners that can be used as substitutes for sugar (pages 3–4).

      b. Name some nutritious substitutes for junk food and drinks (page 4).

      c. What substitutes can you use for salt (page 4)?

      d. Name five of the worst offenders you must omit, once you have made a commitment, (page 5)

      e. Name the kinds of nonprofessional help you can seek (page 5).

   B. *Allergies and the Hyperactive Child*

      1. Philosophy and Scope of Environmental Illness. Chapters 1, 2, 3, and Appendix B, read the following:

      a. Make a list of any of your symptoms that occur in the Allergic-Tension Fatigue Syndrome (pages 4–6).

      b. What is hyperactivity? Are you a hyperactive adult? List your symptoms (pages 23–26).

      c. Do you have an allergic face? List your symptoms (pages 60–66).

      d. From the chart on pages 66–68, make a list of the symptoms you have.

      e. From Appendix B, pages 126–127, read the list of "Medical Problems and Possible Major Food and Other Suspects." Make a list of which, if any, apply to you.

      2. Optional Reading

   "Food for Thought," pages 108–118

Class One

PREVIEW

As you have noticed in the Table of Contents, this book is
organized into "classes." Together the classes become a
course of study. As with most educational programs, textbooks
play a role in your course of environmental medicine.
Before each class there are prescribed readings from the
student/patient textbooks. There are assignments in the
form of key questions and instructions to the reader. The
authors point out the importance of continuing education in
the subject and how attitude plays an important role in
successfully completing this course and in achieving good
health.

OBJECTIVES OF THE COURSE

In many ways environmental medicine is the enlightened
approach to good health. The cost of health services is
constantly spiraling upward, specialized care may be beyond
the geographic if not financial reach of many, and medical
care is frequently provided without education for maintaining
good health—these are but some of the problems addressed
by environmental medicine. Living well can be easier, less
expensive, and available for all, if courses such as this one
are available. These, then, are the goals of environmental
medicine. The following objectives of this course when met
should make these goals attainable. This course will:

1 Serve as an introduction to environmental medicine and its
philosophy.

2 Help you recognize environmental illness in yourself and others.

3 Help you cut down the cost of consultation with your physician,
put you in control of your own health and free your doctor for
medical rather than educational problems.

4   Give you the knowledge of the most common antigens (irritants) in order to prevent or alleviate chemical susceptibility.

5   Serve as a reference for future procedures and purchases of many foods and common household goods.

6   Provide you with the knowledge to educate others who are unfamiliar with the clinical ecologist's approach to medicine.

7   Teach you to cope with all kinds of stress, especially the stress of allergens and pollutants in your environment.

Objectives of Each Class

At the beginning of each class you will find its objectives. Read them carefully at least twice. Read them before you begin the class so you will know what to expect. After you have finished each class go back to reread its objectives in order to evaluate your own progress.

Course Design

The course is designed to be taken in two ways. The first is in the traditional classroom setting under the direction of a counselor appointed by a clinical ecologist who is a medical doctor specializing in environmental medicine. The second way to take this course is at home. If you plan to take the course at home (under the supervision of a doctor), turn to Part II and Part III for further guidance. If you have further questions, consult with your physician's staff member who is supervising your education.

Part III of this book, "Lesson Plans," is important to patients, but it was written expressly to guide the counselor who is conducting this course in the traditional classroom manner. There is a direct correlation between counselor instructions and specific classes that *all* patients/students will participate in. If you are taking this course at home, therefore, you may very well benefit from the information in Part III. A word of caution: read the class sections *and* the corresponding counselor sections *in sequence as you progress in the course.* Do not skip around, unless specifically directed by the author to consult another part of this book

The organizing feature of this course no matter where it is taken is the guided readings from six prescribed books. You will note that some of the books are available in both hard cover and paperback editions (which are revised, updated versions). Page references for assigned readings are given for both editions for readers who already own the hardcover books. The letters "H" and "P" following the page assignments differentiate the editions.

1 Crook, William, M.D. *The Yeast Connection.* Jackson, Tennessee: Professional Books, 1983 (Hardcover), 1988 (Paperback)

Crook discusses the relationship role of yeast/mold sensitivities with environmental illness.

2 Golos, Natalie and Frances Golos Golbitz. *Coping With Your Allergies.* New York: Fireside, 1986. (Paperback)

The authors have written a comprehensive, practical guide and reference book that teaches you how to live with and control your allergies.

or

Golos, Natalie and Frances Golos Golbitz. *Coping With Your Allergies.* New York: Simon and Schuster, 1979. (Hardcover)

3 Golos, Natalie and Frances Golos Golbitz. *If This Is Tuesday, It Must be Chicken.* New Canaan, Connecticut: Keats Publishing, Inc., 1981, 1983. (Paperback)

The authors teach you how to rotate your food for better health.

4 Levin, Alan Scott, M.D. and Merla Zellerbach. *The Type 1/Type 2 Allergy Relief Program.* Los Angeles: Jeremy P. Tarcher, Inc., 1983. Distributed by Houghton Mifflin Company, Boston. (Hardcover).

5 Randolph, Theron G., M.D. and Ralph Moss, Ph.D. *An Alternative Approach to Allergies.* New York: Bantam Books, 1982. (Paperback)

or

Randolph, Theron G., M.D. and Ralph Moss, Ph.D. *An Alternative Approach to Allergies.* New York: Lippincott and Crowel, 1980. (Hardcover)

The authors provide an understanding of the philosophy and distinctive features of clinical ecology and ways of applying the information to your own needs.

6 Rapp, Doris J., M.D. *Allergies and the Hyperactive Child.* New York: Cornerstone Library, 1980. (paperback)

Dr. Rapp provides an overview of the subject of allergies by answering the most frequently asked questions. Dr. Rapp's answers apply to health problems of adults as well as children.

Assignments

The class assignments are divided into four categories:

1 Questions that provoke your thinking and lead you to the books where you will find the answers and stimulate your curiosity for more information.

2 Questions that teach you how to make use of the information and apply it to your individual health needs.

3 Papers for your study that were written specifically for this course.

4 Tests to supplement those done by your doctor.

Importance of Attitude

This course offers hope to those whose doctors for years have been unable to diagnose their chronic illness. For those who know they have mild allergies, it offers a formula for preventing the escalation of their problems. For the health oriented, it offers a word of caution, *prevention*. Since there is a tendency for allergies or immune sensitivities in some families, this message of prevention is of particular importance to the healthy members of any family that includes an allergic person.

At first introduction to the literature, the scope of the problem and the procedures for dealing with it may appear overwhelming. Don't panic! It appears overwhelming only because all degrees of the illness are being addressed in an effort to cover every situation. If you are not severely sensitive, by begining now, you have the advantage of selecting a modified program.

Don't try to be a "100 percenter!" Our environment is so contaminated that even the most sensitive patient can't achieve perfection in avoiding such contamination. Where man has not polluted, nature frequently has. So, do not try the impossible. Don't say, "I can't do it all, so I'll forget it." Be selective now while you still have the choice. The keynote to prevention as well as to management of allergies, mild and complex, is education. Proper education will enable you to make the right choices.

Importance of Education

Education in environmental medicine is as important for the child or the teenager as it is for the adult. One cannot begin too early to develop respect for the environment and vigilance about its pollution. To gain the utmost in cooperation, read the assignments as a family project, doing a couple of sections at a time. Before reading a section, read the assignment questions aloud. See who, if anyone, knows the answers. Then have someone read the sections aloud. As the group searches for the answers, individuals will find additional facts that will very likely apply to some of the "healthy" family members.

Many families who have tried this have reported surprising results after five or six weeks. They have noted the improvement of the allergic patient and also improvement of the health of the so-called "healthy" members. By correcting the diet and other elements of the environment, families have noticed positive changes in personality and interpersonal relationships. They have seen greater energy among family members and improvement in their general wellbeing. They have been grati· fied with the diminished irritability of family members as wel as their relief from minor headaches and other pains.

There is another aspect to the importance of education iı the field of environmental medicine. Although a good deal ha been written on the subject, as the bibliography for this boo attests, dissemination of information is slow. The many wh have been helped with their allergy problems want others ı benefit from the approach of the clinical ecologist. It is impo. tant, therefore, to help create a demand for the availability of well-written materials in your public library.

Requests for such books are what libraries need to hear in order to know what to purchase for their shelves. Of course, more people than the library staff will benefit from this. The person who is merely browsing in material on healthful living will profit as much as the reader who is looking for specific material on environmental medicine. In the long run, the more people who are educated in this field, the greater will be the consumer demand for protection. Also, the greater will be the chances of all to live normal lives.

Some Brief Definitions

You would not be reading a book on healthy living if you were not interested in better health. You would not be reading this book unless you were especially interested in the environment and its effect on human health. Specifically, you are interested in allergies and sensitivities and what can be done about them.

Various readings from the prescribed texts will develop the concepts necessary for educating yourself about environmental medicine. But, it may be useful to review briefly a few fundamental definitions

■ Adaptability: the body's ability to adjust to foreign substances.

■ Allergy: a condition of altered reactivity to a substance which is generally considered benign.

■ Chemical susceptibility: A condition characterized by adverse reaction to concentrations of chemicals generally considered tolerated.

■ Clinical ecologist: a physician who practices clinical ecology.

■ Clinical ecology: a medical discipline in which environmental causes of illness are uncovered and treated.

■ Food addiction: a condition characterized by the dependence of a certain food which produces withdrawal symptoms if the food is not eaten.

■ Masked sensitivity: a condition characterized by a chronic illness which resolves when an individual discontinues exposure to a substance (food, chemical or drug) which appeared to be well tolerated.

■ Food sensitivity: the inability to tolerate certain foods.

■ Withdrawal: (pertaining to illness arising for a short time after terminating exposure to a substance) the unpleasant group of symptoms associated with removal of a food or chemical to which a person is addicted.

And so, armed with some definitions and a relatively new vocabulary of terms, you are ready to see how and why *temporary relief hides the symptoms of disease.* Awareness of the potential changes and side effects of medicines that hide symptoms will be one result of your study. The environmental approach to your well being will help you see that many chronic illnesses *can be reversed.* Good living habits, perhaps new to you, will be emphasized throughout this course. Feeding, bathing, cleaning practices that will tidy up your environment (your food, water, and air) give you the assurance of healthier, happier years.

Precautions

If you have not already done so, this is a good tme for you to start developing sound ecologic habits. It will insure greater accuracy for your testing. You can begin with the following precautions:

FOODS

- Eat no food prepared with additives, preservatives, or artificial food coloring.
- Eliminate junk food and sugars from the diet.
- Use bottled or filtered water, in glass containers only.
- Use fresh or frozen food, avoiding canned food.

FABRICS

- When possible, choose natural fabrics, such as cotton, wool, linen and silk.
- If you can not find natural fabrics, use blends of at least 60% cotton.
- Choose nylon, dacron, and polyester in that order, but only as a last resort.

PERSONAL CARE SUPPLIES

- Use unscented products. This would include bath soaps, shampoos, cosmetics, and deodorants. Use *no* perfume, cologne, or toilet water.
- Use natural toothpaste and a natural bristle toothbrush, a natural bristle hair brush, and a stainless steel or wooden comb.

LAUNDRY SUPPLIES

- Avoid scented laundry soaps, anti-static agents, and fabric softeners.

PAPER PRODUCTS

- Use unscented, white facial tissue and bathroom tissue paper.

PURCHASES

- Check labels on all purchases. Choose products that are less toxic. If a product has a strong odor, do not purchase it.

■ Do not buy products in aerosol cans. "hypoallergenic" usually means synthetic and, therefore, products so labeled are not acceptable.

PERSONAL HEALTH CARE

■ Get adequate rest.

■ Exercise *at least* thirty minutes per day: walking, jogging, bicycling, or other exercise with your doctor's approval.

If you are at home, taking this course under the supervision of a doctor, turn to Part III, Class One lesson plan for further guidance. If you still have questions, consult with the physician's staff member who is supervising your education.

ASSIGNMENT FOR CLASS TWO

I. Read Class Two and be prepared to discuss food sensitivity and the Rotary Diversified Diet.

   A. Begin preparing a list of ways you intend to save money the healthy way.

   B. Make a list of the yeast and mold foods you will begin to eliminate from your diet.

II. *If This Is Tuesday, It Must Be Chicken*

   A. Rotating foods

Read: Chapters 3 and 4

      1. Name one reason for rotating foods.

      2. Name one advantage of rotating foods.

   B. Food families

See: Appendix A.

      1. In the alphabetical list on page 100, what are the first two foods beginning with "b"? You will note that they are "baker's yeast" and "bamboo shoots."

      2. Turn to the numerical list on page 109. Using the numbers for "baker's yeast" and "bamboo shoots," find their food families. Name two more foods in each family.

      3. Using the alphabetical list beginning on page 100, find the number of the food family of your favorite vegetable. Then turn to the numerical list to find what other foods are in that family.

      4. Familiarize yourself with the two lists by finding other foods.

      5. Write an alphabetical list of all your known food allergens (the foods to which you are allergic). Refer to the alphabetical list and write the number before each food you find in the list. Bring two copies of your list to class.

III. *Allergies and the Hyperactive Child*

Read: Appendix B-15

Note the prescription drugs that contain yeast or yeastlike substance.

IV. Optional Reading

   A. *If This Is Tuesday, It Must Be Chicken*

      1. Read Chapter 5, "Cooking Hints for the Allergic."

      2. Read Chapter 6, "Making Rotation Work."

   B. *An Alternative Approach to Allergies*

Read Chapter 21, "Clinical Ecology Versus Conventional Medicine."

Class Two

PREVIEW

The fundamental difference between the clinical ecologist and the traditional doctor is that the clinical ecologist recognizes that many chronic illnesses are caused by chemical susceptibilities and food sensitivities; the traditional doctor does not. The rotation diet is an excellent way to alert one to problem foods and to maintain high nutritional standards. Yeast is a particular concern of some food sensitive people and can be avoided. The families of foods are a convenient as well as scientifically sound way of classification for dietary purposes. We can save money because many of the nontoxic products are less expensive than the toxic ones we have been using.

OBJECTIVES

After studying Class Two and its assignment, you should

1 Understand how clinical ecologists differ from traditional doctors.

2 Be familiar with symptoms of environmental illness.

3 Understand the basics of food sensitivity, food addiction, masking, and the Rotary Diversified Diet.

4 Recognize the yeast and mold-containing foods.

5 Know ways to save money while practicing healthful living habits.

6 Understand food families and how they relate to the Rotary Diversified Diet.

Something Is Wrong!

In their earlier work, *Coping With Your Allergies*, the authors describe the clinician's approach to diagnosis. "Over fifty years old, clinical ecology is still called a new approach to medicine. It is the study of man in his relation to his adaptation to his total environment. Because it is a relatively new approach, foreign to many doctors, and not taught in medical schools, it is often rejected by doctors. Patients are often told, 'there is nothing wrong with you ... physically,' implying that their ailment is psychosomatic. All too frequently patients are referred to a psychiatrist in the mistaken belief that their symptoms suggest severe mental disturbance, when in reality the cause is hidden allergies."

Among samples they cite are:

In cases of hyperactive children, or those with learning disabilities, blame is frequently placed upon guilt-ridden parents rather than on the true culprit: hidden allergies and sensitivities. The comment is often made, "There is nothing wrong with the child; perhaps it is the parent." Yet in many cases these conditions are symptomatic of an illness referred to as "chemical susceptibility" or "cerebral food allergy."

Physicians who are not yet educated to an understanding of the practices of clinical ecology frequently are baffled by various chronic illnesses, unaware that some patients should be tested in relation to environmental factors. If there is any persistent or recurrent condition still unresolved by the attending physician, it is recommended that a clinical ecologist be consulted.

Another indication of the need for such consultation is when the symptoms fall into recognizable patterns: Do the symptoms increase at a particular time of day? Or season of the year? Do they increase during a pollution alert? After eating? After shopping? While traveling? During work hours? At school? Such recurring symptoms should be viewed as clues to possible environmental causes.

Sometimes people are too busy to pay attention to what they consider minor problems. Or they may have been so brainwashed about psychosomatic illness that they dismiss minor isolated discomfort, having been taught that it is a sign of courage and strength of character to "grin and bear it." There is nothing courageous about ignoring pain and discomfort.

Allergists and Clinical Ecologists

Before we continue, it may be helpful to understand the differences and similarities between the conventional allergist and the clinical ecologist. Later in this course, this will be covered in greater detail in *Type 1/Type 2 Allergy Relief Program* by Alan Scott Levin, M.D. and Merla Zellerbach. In the meantime, here are a few introductory statements quoted from their book:

Basically speaking, the two doctors are not that dissimilar. Both agree that:

Avoidance is the best treatment for all allergies....

Blood tests, as structured today, are mainly unreliable but can be useful when nothing else is available.

Immunotherapy—building up the immune system with antigens so that the body's own defenses can withstand allergens—is the best treatment after avoidance....

But the doctors also have their disagreements. Conventionalists believe in using drugs and medication as an adjunct to immunotherapy. Clinical ecologists believe medication should be a last resort....

... conventional allergists rarely treat chemical allergies or even acknowledge that they are more than occasional irritants to the skin and respiratory system.

Be warned that your family doctor may not be familiar with the principles of clinical ecology and may be reluctant to recommend this alternative....

If he becomes impatient or angry, is closed to new ideas, or offers to send you to a psychiatrist, find a more compassionate family doctor. There is no question that a significant number of patients who suffer mental and behavioral symptoms would benefit from astute psychiatric treatment, but many of these patients would benefit even more from proper allergy treatment.

Symptoms of Ecologic Illness

Environmental factors have been identified as causes of many forms of acute, chronic, and recurrent illness. Do you suffer from one or more of the following symptoms?

- Itching, flushing, burning or blistering of the skin?
- Fatigue, dizziness, numbness?

■ Blurred vision, headaches, mental depression, poor concentration, behavior changes?

■ Palpitations or skipped heartbeats?

■ Excessive hunger, compulsive eating, or great thirst?

■ Compulsive smoking?

■ Stammering, stuttering, or hoarseness?

■ Health problems such as arthritis, colitis, dermatitis, hypertension, migraine, obesity, alcoholism, epilepsy, colic, hives, urethral or bladder disorders, reading or writing disabilities, gastrointestinal disturbances or psoriasis?

This is only a partial listing of symptoms and health problems frequently related to allergy. This is not to imply that these conditions always are allergy related. But in many cases, they have been eliminated by removing the offending substances from the diet, from the water supply, or from the indoor or outdoor environment. Any tissue, organ or body system can be affected.

An incredible variety of *reversible* physical and mental disturbances can be caused by reactions to commonly encountered and generally unsuspected factors in the environment. Such symptoms and ailments may require the skillful services of a professional who practices clinical ecology.

Food Sensitivity

When you first read about the Rotary Diversified Diet it may sound complicated. However, as you read the cause and effect of food sensitivity, it will give you the incentive to begin making the necessary changes.

To understand food sensitivity, you must know about food addiction and masking. *Coping with Your Allergies* by Golos and Golbitz explains them.

FOOD ADDICTION   It can take up to four days to clear the food from the body including the gastrointestinal tract and other parts of the food absorption system. If you eat a particular food too frequently your system is never free from that food and you can become addicted to it in the same way that one becomes addicted to drugs. The treachery of food addiction is that you can become a food addict and not know it. The reason for that is the problem known as masking.

MASKING Let's assume you are allergic to peanuts. If for a period of ten days you avoid peanuts and everything made with them, you will probably have a very definite reaction shortly after reintroducing them into your diet. Delayed reaction can occur up to eighteen hours after eating.

If you keep on eating peanuts every day, you will have continuing reactions to a lesser degree. Soon you may not notice any reaction at all. This does not mean that you are no longer bothered by peanuts. The symptoms have merely been masked—hidden so they are no longer associated with the food that caused them. Other symptoms may appear; chronic ailments may develop. Eventually you may find that the only time you feel relief from certain complaints is after you have eaten peanuts. You begin to eat peanuts more and more often. When the problem reaches an acute state, you begin to crave them.

The cycle involved is very similar to drug addiction, with two additional problems that make the offender even more difficult to pinpoint. First, peanut oil is used in preparing many foods, so you are not always aware when peanuts are introduced into your system. Second, and even more confusing, is the fact that you may be addicted, in varying degrees, to several foods at once. The picture becomes so muddled that only an experienced clinician can solve the riddle.

Food addiction has been linked so often to schizophrenia, alcoholism, obesity, arthritis, and other disturbances, that we wonder why it is not common practice to pursue the rotary diversified diet as the first step in the treatment of these and other ailments.

ROTARY DIVERSIFIED DIET The rotary diversified diet was devised by the late Dr. Herbert J. Rinkel, and those who have been helped to lead a normal life because of it are greatly indebted to him.

What is the rotary diet? It is an approach to eating that can prevent food allergies and addictions. It is a diet that can be used as a technique for uncovering and diagnosing food allergies and addictions. And finally it is a diet one can use for a short time or for the rest of one's life to treat food allergies and addictions.

Variables to Consider

In discussing food allergies, the authors of *An Alternative Approach to Allergies*, Randolph and Moss, say:

Basically, there are two kinds of food allergies—fixed and nonfixed, or temporary. A fixed allergy is one with which you are probably born, which does not go away with time. These are relatively less common. More frequently, patients can regain tolerance to troublesome foods after a period of some months of avoidance. The greater the reaction to a food, the longer it takes, in general, to reestablish tolerance. The process usually takes from two to eight months, after which the food can usually be eaten again, if used in rotation. Since the incriminated food is often a favorite and is craved in an addictive manner, the hope of regaining tolerance to it offers some consolation to the patient suffering its temporary loss.

The following outline contains a number of relevant topics that can be discussed in connection with the content of all the following classes. Again, you can not be a 100 percenter with these topics—knowledge and understanding will come with progress in the course.

VARIABLES TO CONSIDER
(IN PLANNING A ROTARY DIVERSIFIED DIET)

A. Purpose of the Diet
  1. Prevention
  2. Diagnosis
  3. Treatment
  4. Maintenance
B. State of Health of the Individual
  1. The mildly sensitive individual
  2. A member of the family prone to allergies
  3. The patient with food allergies
  4. The patient with multiple sensitivities (to food, inhalants, chemicals, etc.)
  5. Varying degrees of recovery
C. Degree of Sensitivity
  1. Number of food allergies
  2. Degree of reactions
  3. Degree of other sensitivities (to inhalants, chemicals, etc.)
D. Degree of Cooperation of the Patient
  1. Mother, or other family member, trying to change the diet of the whole family

2. Patient unconvinced of allergies and thus making gradual changes
3. Convinced patient but very addicted or very undisciplined and thus making gradual changes
4. Patient so ill that he will try anything and thus make immediate and comprehensive changes

Beginning Rotation

Some people begin rotating their food even before their first consultation with the doctor. The following plans have been helpful to them.

First, you could use the sample diet (found on the following two pages) which divides foods into four days making sure that all food families are placed on the same day. Other people find it easier to use chapters 7, 8, 9 and 10 of *If This is Tuesday, It Must Be Chicken.*

Using a four-day-plan, the authors prepared food charts, menus and recipes for each day of the four day cycle. For example, all foods, menus and recipes in Chapter 7 are to be used on the first day of every four day cycle. This plan will insure that you are rotating foods properly.

THIS DOES NOT REPLACE THE NEED OF AN INDIVIDUAL DIET PRE-PARED BY A PROFESSIONAL.

If you are avoiding or decreasing your intake of yeasts and molds, you can still use the sample diet or the charts. All you have to do is avoid the recipes that call for yeast and mold foods.

Yeasts

Because yeasts and molds can cause considerable discomfort to food sensitive individuals, yeast and molds are frequently overlooked as sources of allergies because they are not recognized in the particular food source.

Even though you are not allergic to wheat, you may still

Sample Diet

	Day 1	Day 2	Day 3	Day 4
Protein	*All red meats and their products* Beef, veal, lamb, buffalo, goat. Pork. Venison. Milk, yogurt, all cheeses.	*All fish* Haddock, cod, Perch, Carp. Tuna, mackerel. Rock cod. Turbot, sole, halibut, flounder. Trout, salmon. Sardines, herring. Red snapper.	*Fowl and eggs* Chicken, pheasant, guinea hen. Turkey, goose, duck. Eggs.	*Shellfish* Clams, oysters. Crab, shrimp, lobster. Snails, squid. Scallops. Abalone.
Vegetables	Squash, zucchini, pumpkin, cucumber. Mushrooms. Sweet potatoes. Water chestnuts.	Lettuce, artichokes, dandelions, endive. Cabbage, broccoli, turnips, radishes, cauliflower, kohlrabi, rutabaga, Brussels sprouts, mustard greens, kale. Yams, yuca.	All peas and beans, lentils, soy, alfalfa sprouts, bean sprouts (legumes). Carrots, celery, parsnips, parsley. Asparagus, onions, leeks.	Potatoes, tomatoes, eggplant, peppers. Spinach, beets, Swiss chard. Okra. Corn, bamboo shoots.
Fruit	Peaches, apricots, nectarines, cherries, plums, prunes. All melons. Pineapple. Dates.	Bananas. Grapes, raisins. Blueberries, cranberries, huckleberries. Persimmons. Guavas.	Apples, pears. Strawberries, raspberries, blackberries, boysenberries. Papayas. Rhubarb. Mangoes. Currants.	Oranges, grapefruit, lemons, tangerines, kumquats. Avocado. Pomegranates. Figs. Gooseberries.

Seeds and Nuts	Brazil nuts. Filberts, hazelnuts, chestnuts. Pine nuts.	Peanuts, soy nuts. Cashews, pistachios. Sesame seeds.	Pecans, walnuts. Sunflower seeds.	Almonds. Pumpkin seeds. Macadamia nuts.
Other	Wheat, rye, barley, cornmeal, popcorn, cane, oats, rice, millet. Olives.	Buckwheat. Sesame meal. Peanut butter.	Sunflower meal. Tapioca.	Yeast. Coconut. Arrowroot starch. Gelatin.
Sweeteners	Avocado honey.* Molasses, malt syrup.	Clover honey.* Buckwheat honey.*	Maple sugar or syrup. Sage honey.*	Date sugar. Whey, lactose.
Fats and Oils	Corn oil. Cottonseed oil. Olive oil.	Peanut oil, soy oil. Sesame oil. Chicken fat, turkey fat.	Safflower oil, sunflower oil. Walnut oil. Any fish oils.	Butter, lard, beef fat. Almond oil. Coconut oil.
Herbs and Spices	Chili, pimiento, paprika, cayenne, red pepper. Cinnamon, bay leaf.	Garlic, chives. Ginger, cardamon, turmeric. Dill, fennel, caraway, anise, chervil, cumin, coriander.	Mint, sage, rosemary, basil, marjoram, oregano, thyme. Mustard, horseradish. Cream of tartar. Allspice, cloves.	Black pepper. Nutmeg, mace. Vanilla bean.
Teas	Juniper berry. Comfrey. Hops. Sassafras.	Parsley, Alfalfa. Papaya leaf. Senna. Sarsaparilla.	Chamomile, goldenrod. Blueberry. Mint.	Rosehips.

*Honey can be used only once in four days.

become ill after eating bread, the culprit very likely being yeast. Some people can drink milkshakes but are allergic to malted milkshakes. Others have no reaction to a meat gravy, but become ill if there are mushrooms (a mold food) in it.

YEAST ADDITIVES The following foods contain yeast as an additive ingredient in preparation (often called leavening or baker's yeast):

- Breads: light bread, hamburger buns, hotdog buns, rolls (homemade or canned), crackers, pretzels, canned icebox biscuits.
- Pastries: cookies, pies, cakes.
- Flour enriched with vitamins from yeast.
- Milk fortified with vitamins from yeast.
- Meat fried in cracker crumbs or flour.

Pancakes, waffles, muffins, cornbread, and biscuits made with baking powder or soda can be substituted for baker's yeast products. Unbleached 100 percent whole-wheat crackers (matzos) are available for people who can eat wheat but not yeast.

YEAST-FORMING SUBSTANCES The following foods contain yeast or yeastlike substances, because of their nature or the nature of their manufacture or preparation (including brewer's and distiller's yeast and malt):

- Vinegars (apple, pear, grape, and distilled), either used as such or in the preparation of catsup, mayonnaise, salad dressings, barbecue sauce, tomato sauce, sauerkraut, horseradish, pickles, olives, mince pie, Gerber's oatmeal, and barley cereal.
- Fermented beverages: whiskey, wine, brandy, gin, rum, vodka, beer, root beer.
- Fruit juices, either canned or frozen. Only home-squeezed are yeast-free.

Freshly squeezed lemon juice can be used in place of vinegar in mayonnaise.

YEAST DERIVATIVES The following contain substances that are derived from yeast or yeastlike substances:

- Vitamin B, whether capsule or tablet; multiple vitamins that contain vitamin B.
- Antibiotics; meat from animals that are fed antibiotics.

MOLD FOODS Mushrooms, truffles, morels.

MOLD-CONTAINING FOODS Buttermilk, cheeses of all kinds, including cottage cheese, cream cheese, sour cream, sour-cream butter, condiments, spices, and dried herbs of all kinds (pepper, cinnamon).

Saving Money

One of the greatest misconceptions about environmental health revolves around economy. Contrary to what the skeptics would have you believe you can save money when you adopt some of the practices for prevention of allergy. These practices cover a large range of day-to-day activities and a significant part of the household budget. Six general areas of daily living are discussed in the following paragraphs. They are cosmetics, cleaning, entertaining, food, gasoline, and packaging. In the recommended readings you will be introduced to other healthful practices that save money.

Cosmetics

Cosmetics have become part of our way of life. Millions of dollars are spent, you might even say wasted, on cosmetics and toiletries. The reason the money is wasted is that nature provides many inexpensive, natural products that are excellent substitutes for cosmetics. For example, a slice of cucumber rubbed over your face is an excellent astringent. To cleanse your face and tighten the skin, you can rub part of an egg white on your face, leave it on for about thirty minutes (an hour if you have the time), then rinse it off with plain water. You will never find as inexpensive a cleansing face-mask as this. The unused portion of the white from the egg, as well as the yolk, may be added to your next omelet. For more ideas, see Chapter 28 *Of Coping With Your Allergies.*

Cleaning

Some commercials advocate using certain cleaning products because they contain borax. Why not use pure borax? It is a natural mineral with a naturally sweet scent. Dr. Laurence D. Dickey, a pioneer clinical ecologist, has this to say about the use of borax:

For almost ten years, between March 1966 and December 31, 1975, I carried out a hospital comprehensive environmental control program in evaluating patients with ecologic illness. This was accomplished in rooms made as chemically clean as possible. In addition to fixtures and furnishings that were free of plastics and other materials that were known to "gas out," the cleaning compounds were restricted to borax and baking soda. The floors were wet-mopped with borax and filtered water. From February 15, 1972 on, the program was carried on in four especially constructed rooms with their own air-conditioning system separate from the rest of the hospital. This was the Poudre Valley Memorial Hospital Environmental Care unit. Control of chemical contaminates was much easier in this unit.

Bacterial contamination in the past has been a problem in hospitals, and in ours, like others, the pathology department would periodically run culture checks in various areas of the hospital. The hospital pathologist found the rooms we used and the unit never failed any of their routine checks. We felt this very significant since none of the potent phenolic antiseptics were used in our area that were used in the rest of the hospital. It was a common observation that patients often had an adverse chemical reaction if they had occasion to leave the unit and enter the hospital proper.

Borax is good deodorant, mold retardant and evidently a good bacteriostatic agent.

A good way to save money with any kind of soap that you might use is to keep it on a metal stand rather than in a soap dish. In a soap dish, the water collects, leaving the soap to dissolve and get slimy. On the soap stand, the soap rests on metal bars, allowing any water to drip off the soap. Keep a dish under the stand to catch the soapy drippings, and use a sponge to clean out the dish; then use the soapy sponge to clean other surfaces. This represents a saving, however small. Also, when you reach the end of the bar of soap, where all you have left is a sliver, moisten a new bar of soap and the leftover sliver and press them together. They will stick to each other if allowed to stand for a while. On a daily or even weekly basis, these savings can add up quickly.

Entertaining

There are ways to conserve on the cost of entertaining while at the same time curtailing your indoor pollution. For example, many people use chafing dishes that are kept warm by Sterno, a toxic product and one which has to be replaced from time to time. An electric Salton Tray can be used instead of Sterno and in a variety of ways. If the dish you are serving requires a bowl for sauce or gravy, set the bowl of heated food on the tray. It will stay warm. If the food is composed of individual pieces, with no sauce or gravy involved, the pieces of food can be placed directly on the tray after they are cooked, and the tray will keep the food warm. You don't have to have a party to make use of the Salton Tray. You will find it handy for keeping dishes hot at the table for daily use.

Food

In spite of all the talk that natural food and organic food are expensive, you will find that your food costs are less when you practice prevention. The money that you save by avoiding junk foods alone will astonish you. If the children ask for a junk-food snack, compromise by giving them homemade popcorn. Healthful, inexpensive snacks include fruits in season, Spanish peanuts, sunflower seeds, pumpkin seeds, and raisins. None of these costs as much as candies and cookies. Instead of un-healthy, expensive soft drinks, substitute natural, unsweetened fruit juices.

Another way to save money and to practice prevention is to avoid prepackaged foods. Cutting down or eliminating prepackaged foods is like finding a money tree growing in your kitchen.

While fruits and vegetables can be costly in winter, you can learn to buy in quantity when they are in season and less expensive. Prepare them, using handy hints that will save you time as well as money. For example, you may be able to buy apples and pears by the bushel in the fall. Become familiar with what is abundant at specific times of the year in your region. Very often, at the height of the season, farmers will have a minimal charge for fruits and vegetables if you pick or gather them yourself. There are also many places in the country where blackberries and other fruits grow wild. Many families have found they are able to afford even the more costly organic produce by gathering their own. They make a family outing of this activity.

Cookbooks and books about freezing foods often fail to mention many shortcuts that you can use to help avoid the lengthy processing that is accepted practice. For example, if you free one shelf of your freezer, you can freeze an entire bushel of peaches in a few hours. The procedure is to wash the fruit carefully, put them on a towel to absorb excess moisture, then using a cookie sheet or a Pyrex cake dish, place them on the fast-freeze shelf. Once every hour, for the first four hours, separate the peaches with a spatula to make sure that the bottom layer does not adhere to the dish. Leave the peaches in the freezer overnight. The next morning place them in a cellophane bag and return them to the freezer.

When you are ready to eat the peaches, take out as many as you wish and partially defrost them, just enough to enable you to cut through to the pit in wedges. Most fruits when frozen by this method taste best when partially defrosted. If you wish, the skin can be easily removed when the peach is just beginning to defrost. When totally defrosted, it is much better to use the peaches as a puree on cereal, or served with nuts. Some people have to acquire a taste for fruit that is totally defrosted. The reason this freezing method is far superior is that the only time invested is for washing and drying. Fruits that can be frozen whole are:

apples	cherries	pears
apricots	grapes	persimmons
bananas	peaches	plums
berries		

Bananas can be frozen with or without the skin. If you freeze them without the skin, they must be in a tightly-sealed package. Fresh pineapple freezes well if peeled, cut into small wedges, and placed in jars.

Since the heating process needed for canning destroys some of the nutritional value, canning should be done only if there is a shortage of freezer space. Many people resort to drying their foods, but here again the process requires a certain amount of heat and is acceptable though not preferred. Remember: dried food is not acceptable for people with mold and yeast sensitivities.

Many vegetables can be prepared for cooking (washed, dried, sliced, cubed, etc.), placed in a single layer on a cookie sheet, and frozen quickly. As soon as they are frozen, place them in a suitable container and return them to the freezer for use as needed. It is then convenient to grab a handful for use in soups, stews, salads, pot roast, or as garnishes. They do not require blanching before freezing. This processing has worked well with the following vegetables:

carrots (sliced)	green peppers	peas
celery (chopped)	herbs (chopped)	rhubarb
celery leaves (chopped)	onions	shell beans
chives (chopped)	parsnips	squash
corn (removed from cob)		

To dry herbs without losing nutrients, place them in the oven on "warm" (under 140°F.) for several hours or overnight.

For further information about preparing foods, see Chapter 15, "Cooking in Large Quantities," of *Coping With Your Allergies*.

Gasoline

The gasoline pump has an automatic shut-off mechanism when your tank has reached full capacity. After it clicks, the attendant often hand pumps more gasoline, frequently filling your tank beyond its capacity, causing overflow, costing you more money and wasting energy. The next time you are in a gas station, notice the cars pulling away and see the overflow dripping from the cars. This practice incidentally also contributes to the pollution in the air, inside and outside your car. Ask the attendant to stop at the first "click" and not to "round it off." By telling him that you will pay only for the amount registered at the first click, he will be careful to comply with your instructions.

The practice of letting your motor idle wastes gas, wastes money, and causes pollution. Never leave your motor running while waiting in line for someone or something.

Another terrible waste of money is warming up your motor. We were told that, while this practice was necessary years ago, cars now are equipped with devices that make the warming up practice unnecessary. Instead, start your motor and let it run for just thirty seconds. In cold weather drive slowly for several blocks.

Packaging

The use of glass jars is another ecologic way to save money. Restaurants and schools are a good source of used half-gallon and gallon glass jars. Look for jars that have large openings. You can use these to store vegetables, fruits, and meats that do not fit into the special compartments. You may have to remove one shelf of your refrigerator so that jars will fit, but you will be able to accommodate more fresh fruits and vegetables. One double shelf of a seventeen cubic-foot refrigerator can hold eight one-gallon and two or three half-gallon jugs. You can fit more food in the refrigerator by stacking small packages, small casserole dishes, or quart-size jars on top of the gallon jars. The jars can be washed and reused indefinitely, saving you the cost of plastic bags and other types of food wrappings that leak contaminants into the food.

If you are at home, taking this course under the supervision of a doctor, turn to Part III, Class Two lesson plan for further guidance. If you still have questions, consult with the physician's staff member who is supervising your education.

ASSIGNMENT FOR CLASS THREE

I. Read Class Three and be prepared to discuss it.

II. Fill out the "Chemical Questionnaire" and list how it applies to you.

III. Complete the assigned readings and answer all questions on them.
   A. *Coping With Your Allergies.*
   1. Foreword (P pages 9-11 or H pages 9–11)
   Name four factors which can lower resistance and lead to allergies.
   2. "A note to the Mildly Allergic" (P pages 17–18 or H page 15)
   Name two potential dangers of using non-prescription medicines, such as aspirin, cough medicine, and nasal drops.
   3. Chapter 1 (P pages 21–29 or H pages 19–26)
      a. Compare any of your symptoms with those mentioned in the book and indicate which of them you previously did not associate with allergies.
      b. How do you look for patterns that could indicate allergies?
   4. Chapter 2 (P pages 30–39 or H pages 27–35)
      a. Using coffee, candy, or cigarettes as an example, discuss masking.
      b. Give two examples of food addiction.
      c. Check your eating patterns to see if you might be addicted to some food. Are you addicted to one or more of these: cigarettes, perfumes, medicines, alcohol, or sweets?
      d. How will the knowledge of addiction help you prevent the development of food allergies?

5. Chapter 3 (P pages 40–47 or H pages 36–43)

    a. Describe how knowledge about "overloading" can help you prevent food allergies.

    b. What precautions can an expectant mother take to safeguard her child against allergies?

6. Chapter 4 (P pages 48–53 or H pages 44–48)

Prepare a list of troublemakers you find in your home. List those that you wish to change immediately. List future replacements. List simple substitutions you can make.

7. Chapter 5 (P pages 54–61 or H pages 49–55)

    a. What is orthomolecular medicine (as defined by California law)?

    b. What cerebral (brain) allergy symptoms may mislead a psychiatrist?

8. Chapter 6 (P pages 62–66 or H pages 56–59)

List three cardiovascular disorders that have been linked to allergy.

9. Chapter 7 (P pages 67–80 or H pages 60–72)

    a. Practice breathing exercises several times a day.

    b. Start practicing Phase I.

10. Chapter 24 P pages 227–235 or H pages 206–213

Make a list of your current cleaning products. List those that can be replaced by one or a combination of the following: vinegar, baking soda, borax, or trisodium phosphate.

B. *An Alternative Approach to Allergies*

Chapter 19, P pages 223–226 or H pages 188–200

If you have not already done so, answer the questionnaire, P pages 224–235 or H pages 189–199. It will be best if you fill it out completely before reading any of the interpretive material between the sections.

Class Three

PREVIEW

No product is safe for everyone. This caution cannot be repeated too often for the chemically sensitive person. For the mildly allergic, it warrants consideration as well. Beware of products labeled "NEW" or "IMPROVED." A product once safe does not always remain safe. The additive that "improves" the product is usually a chemical that must be avoided. Most cleaning materials, whether for household or clothing, are sources of toxins. After completing Dr. Randolph's chemical questionnaire we will recognize many ways to prevent or lessen "indoor pollution." Environmental analysis can lead to the reduction of unwanted stress in our lives.

OBJECTIVES

After studying Class Three and its assignment you should:

1   Have a thorough knowledge of Randolph's "Chemical Questionnaire" and how it applies to your state of health.

2   Know the relatively safe methods and products for cleaning clothes, houses, and cars.

3   Understand the concept of allergy prevention.

4   Recognize products that are harmful to *your* health.

5   Know good breathing exercises and begin to practice them.

6   Understand the importance of stress reduction.

The Chemical Questionnaire

It is ironic to hear someone with a cigarette in his hand complaining about the failure of the government to protect us from industrial pollution. Not that the complaints are unjustified but how can a task force, studying the health effects from pollution, do so in a smoke-filled room?

In *An Alternative Approach to Allergies*, Randolph discusses air pollution:

It may have occurred to the reader that air pollution plays a role in the problem of chemical susceptibility. This is true, but not in the way most people suspect. For while it is true that outdoor, or ambient, air pollution is a significant source of exposure, a far greater threat is posed by the presence of indoor, or domiciliary, air pollution.

Indoor air pollution? The term itself is unfamiliar and strange to most people, who tend to think of air pollution solely in terms of smog. Yet the home itself generates combustion products or is directly exposed to them, and many household products give off noxious fumes.

Indoor air pollution is particularly dangerous because exposure to it is so constant. Outdoor air pollution comes and goes; indoor pollution is ever-present, and thus it effects generally remain well hidden.

"The Chemical Questionnaire" that follows is from Chapter 19 of *An Alternative Approach to Allergies* by Randolph and Moss. It was designed to help determine the degree of chemical sensitivity, if any, of patients. According to Dr. Randolph, "The answers to these questions serve as a guide to future therapy and prevention." Therefore, in order to gain the most from the questionnaire, you should answer the entire questionnaire with little or no advance knowledge.

In the book there are sections of explanation between portions of the questionnaire. Do not read these sections until you have completed all questions. You may wish to use a sheet of paper with numbers corresponding to the sections of the questionnaire so that others in the family can use the questionnaire.

Human Ecology and Susceptibility to the Chemical Environment Questionnaire

CHEMICAL ADDITIVES AND CONTAMINANTS OF AIR, FOOD, WATER, DRUGS, AND COSMETICS

Date_____ Name_____ Home Address_____
CIRCLE or FILL IN the following: Sex_____ Age_____

Education		**Marital Status**	**Occupation**_____	
Highest school year:		Single	*Work Region*	**Work Address**
1 2 3 4 5 6 7 8	1 2 3 4	Married	City	Distance from work_____
Elementary	High	Widowed	Suburban	**Travel by:**
1 2 3 4	1 2 3 4	Separated	Small town	Car Train Other_____
College	Graduate	Divorced	Rural	Bus Walking_____

Home

Type	*If multiple dwelling*	*Region*	*Garage*
Single House	What floor?_____	City residential	In separate unattached
Double House	How long have you	City industrial	building
Apartment	lived there?_____	Suburban	With inside passageway
Hotel	_____	Small town	between house & garage
Trailer		Rural	In basement of house

Heating & Ventilation of Home

Type	*Fuel*	*Furnace Location*	*Air Conditioning*	*Kitchen Exhaust Fan*
Electric, heat pump	Electric		Window units	
Electric, radiant	Gas	Basement	Central system	Yes
Hot water or steam	Oil	Main floor	Filters—Oiled	No
Warm air	Coal	Utility room	Unoiled	*Kitchen Door*
Space heaters	Wood	Open	Electrostatic	Usually left open
Fireplaces	Other____	Closed	Activated carbon	Usually closed

Utilities

Range	*Refrigerator Type*	*Food Storage*	*Deep Freeze*	*Clothes dryer*	*Water Heater*
Electric			Electric	Electric	Electric
Gas	Electric	in Glass	Gas	Gas	Gas
Oil	Gas	in enamel ware	Age____	Age____	Part of furnace
Age____	Age____	in plastic			Age____

Furnishings and Household Maintenance

Upholstery Coverings	*Padding*	*Mattresses*	*Pillows*	*Rugs*	*Rug Pads*
Cotton Silk	Cotton	Cotton	Feather	Wool	Plastic
Linen Wool	Hair	Rubber	Rubber	Cotton	Rubber
Synthetic fabrics	Rubber	Plastic covered	Kapok	Synthetic	Hair
Plastic	Other____	Other____	Dacron	Natural fiber	
			Plastic covered	Rubber or	
				Plastic backed	

Curtains	Cleansers	Deodorants & Disinfectants	Laundry		Furniture Polish
Cotton silk	Soap		Soap	Plastic starch	
Wool linen	Detergents	Air wick	Bleaches	Cornstarch	Yes No
Plastic	Scouring pwd.	Lysol	Ammonia	Dryer	Floor Wax
Synthetic	with bleach	Pine-Sol	Detergents	Electric	Yes No
material	Ammonia	Others____		Gas	

Miscellaneous

Insect Control	Drinking Water	Sense of Smell	Ability to Detect Leaking Gas	When Wind is Blowing from Industrial Areas
Sprays	Spring or well	Very acute	Acute	Are your symptoms
Moth Balls	Softened	Normal	Normal or average	increased?
Moth Crystals	Chlorinated	Poor	Poor or absent	Unchanged?
Exterminators	Fluoridated	Absent		

WHAT IS YOUR REACTION TO THE FOLLOWING? Check One:

	Like	Neu-tral	Dis-like	Made sick from
Coal, Oil, Gas, & Combustion Products				
1. Massive outdoor exposures to coal smoke	___	___	___	___
2. Smoke in steam railroad stations, train sheds, and yards	___	___	___	___
3. Smoke from coal burning stoves, furnaces, or fireplaces	___	___	___	___
4. Odors of natural gas fields	___	___	___	___
5. Odors of escaping utility gas	___	___	___	___
6. Odors of burning utility gas	___	___	___	___
7. Odors of gasoline	___	___	___	___
8. Garage fumes and odors	___	___	___	___
9. Automotive or motor boat exhausts..........	___	___	___	___
10. Odor of naphtha, cleaning fluids, or lighter fluids	___	___	___	___
11. Odor of recently cleaned clothing, upholstery, or rugs......................................	___	___	___	___
12. Odor of naphtha-containing soaps	___	___	___	___
13. Odor of nail polish or nail polish remover	___	___	___	___
14. Odor of brass, metal, or shoe polishes	___	___	___	___
15. Odor of fresh newspapers	___	___	___	___
16. Odor of kerosene	___	___	___	___
17. Odor of kerosene or fuel-oil burning lamps or stoves	___	___	___	___
18. Odor of kerosene or fuel-oil burning space heaters or furnaces...........................	___	___	___	___
19. Diesel engine fumes from trains, buses, trucks, or boats....................................	___	___	___	___
20. Lubricating greases or crude oil	___	___	___	___
21. Fumes from automobiles burning an excessive amount of oil				

	Like	Neu-tral	Dis-like	Made sick from
22. Fumes from burning greasy rags	___	___	___	___
23. Odors of smudge pots as road markers or frost inhibitors	___	___	___	___

WHAT IS YOUR REACTION TO THE FOLLOWING? Check One:

	Like	Neu-tral	Dis-like	Made sick from
Mineral Oil, Vaseline, Waxes, & Combustion Products				
1. Mineral oil as contained in hand lotions and medications	___	___	___	___
2. Mineral oil as a laxative	___	___	___	___
3. Cold cream or face or foundation cream	___	___	___	___
4. Vaseline, petroleum jelly, or petrolatum-containing ointments.......................................	___	___	___	___
5. Odors of floor, furniture, or bowling alley wax...	___	___	___	___
6. Odors of glass wax or similar glass cleaners ...	___	___	___	___
7. Fumes from burning wax candles	___	___	___	___
8. Odors from dry garbage incinerators.	___	___	___	___

WHAT IS YOUR REACTION TO THE FOLLOWING? Check One:

	Like	Neu-tral	Dis-like	Made sick from
Asphalts, Tars, Resins, & Dyes				
1. Fumes from tarring roofs and roads	___	___	___	___
2. Asphalt pavements in hot weather	___	___	___	___
3. Tar-containing soaps, shampoos, and ointments	___	___	___	___
4. Odors of inks, carbon paper, typewriter ribbons, and stencils	___	___	___	___
5. Dyes in clothing and shoes....................	___	___	___	___
6. Dyes in cosmetics (lipstick, mascara, rouge, powder, other)	___	___	___	___

WHAT IS YOUR REACTION TO THE FOLLOWING? Check One:

	Like	Neu-tral	Dis-like	Made Sick from
Disinfectants, Deodorants, & Detergents				
1. Odor of public or household disinfectants and deodorants....................................	___	___	___	___
2. Odor of phenol (carbolic acid) or Lysol	___	___	___	___

	Like	Neu-tral	Dis-like	Made sick from
3. Phenol-containing lotions or ointments	___	___	___	___
4. Injectable materials containing phenol as a preservative	___	___	___	___
5. Fumes from burning creosote-treated wood (rail-road ties)....................................	___	___	___	___
6. Household detergents	___	___	___	___

WHAT IS YOUR REACTION TO THE FOLLOWING? *Check One:*

	Like	Neu-tral	Dis-ike	Made sick from
Rubber				
1. Odor of rubber or contact with rubber—gloves, elastic in clothing, girdles, brassieres, garters, etc..	___	___	___	___
2. Odor of sponge-rubber bedding, rug pads, type-writer pads	___	___	___	___
3. Odor of rubber-based paint	___	___	___	___
4. Odor of rubber tires, automotive accessories, etc..	___	___	___	___
5. Odor of rubber-backed rugs and carpets	___	___	___	___
6. Fumes of burning rubber.....................	___	___	___	___

WHAT IS YOUR REACTION TO THE FOLLOWING? *Check One:*

	Like	Neu-tral	Dis-like	Made sick from
Plastics, Synthetic Textiles, Finishes, & Adhesives				
1. Odor of or contact with plastic upholstery, table-cloths, book covers, pillow covers, shoe bags, handbags	___	___	___	___
2. Odor of plastic folding doors or interiors of automobiles	___	___	___	___
3. Odors of or contact with plastic spectacle frames, dentures	___	___	___	___
4. Odor of plastic products in department or spe-cialty stores	___	___	___	___
5. Nylon hose and other nylon wearing apparel ...	___	___	___	___
6. Dacron or Orlon clothing or upholstery	___	___	___	___
7. Rayon or cellulose-acetate clothing or upholstery .	___	___	___	___
8. Odor of or contact with adhesive tape	___	___	___	___
9. Odor of plastic cements	___	___	___	___

WHAT IS YOUR REACTION TO THE FOLLOWING? *Check One:*

	Like	Neu-tral	Dis-like	Made sick from
Alcohols, Glycols, Aldehydes, Ketones, Esters, Terpines, & Derived Substances				
1. Odor of rubbing alcohol	——	——	——	——
2. Alcohols or glycols as contained in medications	——	——	——	——
3. Odor of varnish, lacquer, or shellac	——	——	——	——
4. Odor of drying paint	——	——	——	——
5. Odor of after-shave hair tonics or hair oils	——	——	——	——
6. Odor of window cleaning fluids	——	——	——	——
7. Odor of paint or varnish thinned with mineral solvents.....................................	——	——	——	——
8. Odor of banana oil (amyl alcohol)............	——	——	——	——
9. Odor of scented soap and shampoo	——	——	——	——
10. Odor of perfumes and colognes	——	——	——	——
11. Odor of Spray Net® and other hair dressings..	——	——	——	——
12. Fumes from burning incense	——	——	——	——

WHAT IS YOUR REACTION TO THE FOLLOWING? *Check One:*

	Like	Neu-tral	Dis-like	Made sick from
Miscellaneous				
1. Air conditioning	——	——	——	——
2. Ammonia fumes............................	——	——	——	——
3. Odor of moth balls	——	——	——	——
4. Odor of insect-repellant candles	——	——	——	——
5. Odor of termite extermination treatment	——	——	——	——
6. Odor of DDT-containing insecticide sprays....	——	——	——	——
7. Odor of Chlordane, Lindane, Parathione, Dieldrin, and other insecticide sprays	——	——	——	——
8. Odor of weed killers (herbicides)	——	——	——	——
9. Odor of the fruit and vegetable sections of supermarkets	——	——	——	——
10. Odor of dry goods stores and clothing departments.......................................	——	——	——	——
11. Odor of formalin or formaldehyde	——	——	——	——
12. Odor of chlorinated water	——	——	——	——
13. Drinking of chlorinated water	——	——	——	——
14. Fumes of chlorine gas	——	——	——	——
15. Odor of Clorox and other hypochlorite bleaches.	——	——	——	——
16. Fumes from sulfur processing plants	——	——	——	——
17. Fumes of sulfur dioxide	——	——	——	——

WHAT IS YOUR REACTION TO THE FOLLOWING? *Check One:*

	Like	Neutral	Dislike	Made sick from

Pine

1. Odor of Christmas trees & other indoor evergreen decorations . . . .
2. Odor of knotty pine interiors . . . .
3. Odor from sanding or working with pine or cedar woods . . . .
4. Odor of cedar-scented furniture polish . . . .
5. Odor of pine-scented household deodorants . . .
6. Odor of pine-scented bath oils, shampoos, or soaps . . . .
7. Odor of turpentine or turpentine-containing paints
8. Fumes from burning pine cones or wood . . . . . .

Classes of Drugs, or Drugs—Circle If Suspected

Name Others Not Listed

Analgesics
Androgens
Anesthetics, local
Anesthetics, general
Antibiotics
Anticoagulants
Anticonvulsants
Antihistaminics
Antispasmodics
Asthma remedies
Diuretics
Estrogens
Headache remedies
Laxatives
Opiates
Sedatives
Steroids
Tranquilizers
Vaccines
Vitamins

Adrenalin (epinephrine)
Aminophyllin
Aspirin (Bufferin, Empirin)
Barbiturates
Codeine
Demerol
Ephedrine
Ether
Iodides
Mineral Oil
Morphine
Novocaine
Penicillin
Phenobarbital
Phenolphthalein
Saccharine
Stilbestrol
Sucaryl
Sulfonamides
Vaseline

Drugs Currently Being Used—Circle If Suspected

_____	_____	_____
_____	_____	_____
_____	_____	_____
Currently used Dentifrice	Currently used Mouthwash	Others

Currently used Cosmetics	(name brands, if possible)	
Deodorant_____	**For Women**	**For Men**
Toilet soap_____	Face Powder_____	Electric preshave
Shampoo_____	Dusting Powder_____	_____
Hand Lotion_____	Lipstick_____	After shaving lotion
Cold cream_____	Foundation cream_____	_____
Contraceptive_____	Nail polish_____	Hair Oil_____
_____	Perfume_____	_____
_____	Cologne_____	Others_____
_____	Mascara_____	_____
_____	Eyebrow pencil_____	_____
_____	Cold Wave_____	_____
_____	Permanent_____	_____
	Hair tint_____	
	Douche_____	

Do you smoke . . . cigarettes _____ pipe_____ cigars_____
Age you started to smoke _____ Age you last quit smoking _____
Was it difficult to stop? _____ Number of smokes per day _____
What is your maximum weight?_____ Your present weight? _____

Interpreting the Questionnaire

Now that you have completed the questionnaire you will be able to judge your answers more clearly by turning to Dr. Randolph's book and carefully reading the section that precedes each part. To quote him, "Bear in mind that positive answers on the questionnaire itself only indicate that a problem may exist. They are a good signal to seek further professional help and to institute some preventive techniques. . . ."

To help you better understand the value of the questionnaire, turn to "An Alternative Approach to Allergies" P page 227 or H page 191. Note the section entitled "What is your reaction to the following?" You will see that the main topic is entitled "Coal, Oil, Gas and Combustion Products." It may be obvious to you that the odor of gasoline or garage fumes (No. 7) bothers you. However, you may not recognize a problem resulting from exposure to naptha, cleaning fluids or lighter fluids (No. 10) or, on the next page, soaps (No. 12) or fresh newspapers (No. 15).

Similarly, you may be aware of having a problem with asphalts and tars, listed on P page 229 or H page 193. However, their by-products, such as dyes in cosmetics (No. 6), may escape your notice.

It is therefore very important for you to associate all the by-products with their chemical sources. As you study your answers, if you see that there are certain sections where everything has made you sick, it is obvious that you should consider avoiding these products. Furthermore, it may indicate the need to take preventive measures seriously. In the event that there are several categories that cause you a great deal of trouble, request a private consultation with the doctor, or at least bring it to the attention of the course instructor.

Cleaning

No product is safe for everyone. Before using any new product or process, the chemically-sensitive patient must test it in very small quantities as instructed by his physician.

Most of the cleaning products discussed at length in the assigned reading for this class from *Coping With Your Allergies* are unchanged and still recommended. Therefore, since space is limited, we shall discuss only those that are no longer acceptable, as well as some new products that we find promising.

Products to Avoid

The following products, originally suggested in the hardcover edition of *Coping With Your Allergies*, are no longer satisfactory for sensitive patients:

1   ARM & HAMMER WASHING SODA   This product was once considered relatively safe for the chemically-sensitive patient and was recommended for heavy-duty laundry and cleaning, especially for sink and bathtub drains. Now, however, in some parts of the country, the manufacturers appear to be distributing a changed formula. For the chemically-sensitive, Arm & Hammer Washing Soda is no longer acceptable for clothes and should be used in plumbing only with discretion.

2 BON AMI CLEANING POWDER in the round can contains toxic additives. The Bon Ami Cleaning Powder in the square can *is* still acceptable. It is made of Bon Ami Bar Soap that is finely ground. Both the cleaning powder and the bar soap can be purchased from the manufacturer:

> Faultless Starch/Bon Ami Company
> 1025 West 8th Street
> Kansas City, Missouri 64101
> Telephone: 861–842–2030

They will gladly furnish you with the name of a local distributor or ship directly to you.

3 INFINITY SHAMPOO The label of this product now lists formaldehyde as one of its ingredients. As a general precaution before buying any shampoo, even if you have safely used it in the past, check the label to make sure of its contents. See below for a suggested alternative shampoo.

New Products

Neo-Life Company of America (Hayward, California 94545) man- ufactures many products reputed to be toxic-free. Three of their products appear to be fairly well tolerated by the chemically-sensitive person. These are Organic Green, Rugged Red, and Neo-life dishwashing detergent. Some chemically-sensitive patients have been able to tolerate Mellow Yellow, Plus, and Super Plus, but these products are not advised for the patient with extreme susceptibility. They can, however, serve as a substitute for toxic products in a home where prevention of chemical sensitivities is being practiced. Organic Green and Rugged Red appear to have even wider use than the company recommends.

ORGANIC GREEN Many people have found this product safe for bathing, shampooing hair, brushing teeth, and washing delicate fabrics. It can be used in the washing machine (for heavy-duty laundry add either Borax, Neo-Life Plus, or Super Plus, if toler- ated). Organic Green is also excellent for washing silk clothing. One man has reported that it is an excellent shaving product. Organic Green also makes an excellent insect repellent that works for some people. First, test it on a small area of your wrist, near your pulse. If you do not have a reaction, you can use it liberally. Before going outside into mosquito or gnat infested environments, spread it liberally over all exposed parts of your body, except near your eyes.

RUGGED RED This product is a heavy-duty cleaner. It can be used for cleaning woodwork, appliances, walls, floors, bathrooms, bathroom tile, windows, and cars. It seems to be quite effective as a mold retardant. In addition, it is a good household insect repellent for spider mites, silverfish, and ants. By spraying screens and window sills with Rugged Red, it is possible to repel flies that tend to enter between the window and the screen.

How to Use Bon Ami Bar Soap

Always be sure that the soap bar is on a platform away from water so that it does not soak in water. Appropriate holders are widely available.

Never wet the bar of soap. Always dampen the cloth that you are going to use and rub it on the dry bar. It is more effective this way, and the bar will last for a long time. Bon Ami Bar Soap seems to be expensive, but because it lasts so long it is actually less expensive than most other bar soaps.

Bon Ami Bar Soap is most effective for washing walls. Rub a damp cloth lightly across the bar of soap, and then run the cloth over the area to be cleaned. Follow this first with a slightly damp cloth, then a dry cloth. Unless the wall is extremely soiled, it does not take much pressure to get it clean.

Bon Ami Bar Soap is always very effective for cleaning dirty spots on kitchen and bathroom floors. Usually, the same procedure as that followed for walls is satisfactory. If the floor is very dirty, dampen a pad of the soap free American Steel stainless steel wool, rub it on the soap, scrub the area, and then rinse. It should be noted that Rugged Red is actually the best product to use for floors because it is the easiest. However, for those people who cannot tolerate Rugged Red, the Bon Ami Bar Soap with the steel wool is also satisfactory. The only problem with this procedure is that the Bon Ami may leave a little grit, which must be thoroughly rinsed.

The Bon Ami Bar Soap works well on porcelain, stainless steel, woodwork, and windows. In fact, you can use it for any job for which you would normally use a cleanser.

BON AMI CLEANING POWDER   The Bon Ami in the square yellow box may be easier to use than the bar soap. The powdered cleanser is made of ground-up Bon Ami Bar Soap. To clean an oven, wet the soiled area, pour on dry Bon Ami, heat the oven for twenty minutes at 200 degrees (F.) and then wipe the oven with damp paper towels. If you cannot use paper towels, use damp rags. This may not be so effective as some of the toxic substances that you have used in the past. If you are careful about the buildup of soil in your daily use of the oven, you will find this cleaning method adequate.

The art of maintaining a clean stove is by cooking foods in the most wholesome way. This means that you should:

1   Never heat foods at too high a temperature.
2   Never fry foods.
3   Seldom broil foods.
4   Steam or poach foods as often as possible.

The wisest cooking method is over slow heat for a longer period of time. If you use this procedure and avoid filling the utensil too full, it will curtail spillage and thus avoid tough cleaning jobs. If, in spite of these precautions, you do create a soiled area, clean it up as soon as possible.

The Bon Ami Bar Soap and the Bon Ami Cleaning Powder can be used interchangeably. The one difference is that the powder seems to leave more of a grit and thus takes more effort to rinse. The advantage of the powder, however, is that it is a little easier to use, especially when you have a large area to clean. This, of course, does not apply to walls. Here you should use the bar soap.

How To Use Rugged Red

Whether or not you use Rugged Red depends on the degree of your sensitivity. Put one part Rugged Red and seven parts water in the spray bottle that comes with the purchase. Some patients have reported that they sometimes use a larger ratio of Rugged Red, as much as four parts Rugged Red to four parts water. Some people have found it necessary to soak very soiled areas for an hour or so with a full strength solution.

Spray the Rugged Red solution on the surface that you are cleaning. Rub the surface with a dry cloth, until you get all the dirt off. Then spray the surface a second time and rub it with a clean cloth. The surface does not have to be rinsed. In fact, Rugged Red left on the surface that you have cleaned acts as an excellent insect and mold retardant. Just be sure that your solution is not too concentrated or your surface will be sticky.

Cleaning with Rugged Red will eliminate silverfish if that is a problem, although it will do so only after several applications. You can also spray areas around windows, where there are signs of spider mites. Wipe dry after spraying, and then spray again. Gradually this will help eliminate the insects. In addition to its household uses, Rugged Red is an excellent cleaner for your automobile.

It is worth mentioning that the spray procedure may not be safe for some people. They might be bothered by it, because the spray, which is an atomizer, spreads the Rugged Red directly into the air. If this is a problem, you can make the same mixture and rub it on with a damp cloth. If you cannot stand the direct contact, have someone else do it for you. You may or may not be able to leave some on the surface. It is important to note here that you may not be able to use Rugged Red or other substances unless someone else applies them.

How to Use Organic Green

Organic Green, like all products that you are using for the first time, must be tested from the standpoint of your sensitivity. It is generally more easily tolerated than other cleaning substances and worth trying as a substitute for them.

Organic Green appears to work wonders on even the most delicate fabrics, such as silk clothing. To remove grease from silk clothing, rub a little Organic Green on the spot, let it sit for ten minutes, rinse it off, and then wash the whole garment in Organic Green. You may need to do it a second time, but eventually this treatment should take care of the grease spot even if it has been there for some time.

When washing cotton clothing, rub a little Organic Green under the arms of the garment to remove the salt that remains there from perspiration. Rub it briskly, then dip the garment in water. No additional Organic Green is needed in the water. Rinse twice in clear water. Use the same procedure for the crotch of the underpants or the underarm of your bras. This should be done to any part of a garment that is subject to perspiration or excessive soiling. If you are washing a substantial number of garments at the same time, follow the above procedure but skip the rinsing. Finish the washing process in your machine.

Neolife Dishwashing Detergent

If you can tolerate a dishwasher you may be able to use Neolife dishwashing detergent. This product is less offensive than most commercial products.

When running the dishwasher leave the room. Allow plenty of ventilation in the room where the dishwasher is located. This is necessary because the plastic parts of the dishwasher heat up when the machine is running.

Cautionary Notes

Very often the authors suggest a specific product, because it has been used safely by a number of very sensitive people. In spite of this, there are precautions that should be mentioned. Because some sensitive people can tolerate the product, does not mean that every sensitive person can. Because we suggest some products from a particular company does not mean that all of their products are acceptable. For example, we are enthusiastic about Organic Green, Rugged Red, and the Neolife Dishwashing Detergent, but this does not mean that we recommend the vitamin products distributed by the same company, no matter what they or anyone else might say.

As we have mentioned before, you should test all new products yourself. Do this in the following way. Wash just one item, perhaps a cotton handkerchief. Wash and rinse it carefully, and then try using it. Wash it again and use it. Repeat this process several times. Often people can tolerate a product for a while and then become sensitive to it. This has happened with Borax. Perhaps this happens because some residue frequently remains after rinsing. On the other hand, frequent use may sensitize a person to the product.

If you are at home, taking this course under the supervision of a doctor, turn to Part III, Class Three lesson plan for further guidance. If you still have questions, consult with the physician's staff member who is supervising your education.

ASSIGNMENT FOR CLASS FOUR

I. Read Class Four

    A. Be prepared to discuss the facts you should know about your immune system.

    B. List any questions you have about doing your own testing.

    C. Complete the rest of the assignment before you attempt any tests.

II. Complete the assigned readings and and answer all questions. The assigned readings for Class Four are from *An Alternative Approach to Allergies.*

    A. Chapter 1 P pages 19–35 or H pages 15–28(/)

        1. Using the Addiction Pyramid, name the two most quickly absorbed food ingestants.

        2. Name the two phases of the addictive response.

        3. How did Dr. Herbert Rinkel discover his hidden allergy to eggs and eventually his discovery of food addiction?

    B. Chapter 2 pages 36–48 or H pages 29–39(P/)

        1. Study Table 1, "The Ups and Downs of Addiction." Locate some of your reactions and note the levels on which they occur.

    C. Chapter 8 P pages 139–145 or H pages (/97–100/)

        1. Name three serious medical problems on the Stimulatory Level.

        2. Name the major manifestations of the Minus-Two Level.

    D. Chapter 11 P pages 139–145 or H pages 117–122(/)

        1. Name the six major kinds of localized reactions.

        2. Name five kinds of systemic withdrawal manifestations.

III. Optional Reading

An Alternative Approach to Allergies

Read Chapters 3 through 7 and Chapters 9 through 15.

Class Four

PREVIEW

We now know that chemical sensitivity is a malfunction of the immune system. This condition can be improved by a comprehensive health program. Prevention is the least expensive way to cope with a medical problem. Hand in hand with preventive measures goes the concept of self-testing, for one must know what is affecting one's state of health.

OBJECTIVES

After studying Class Four and its assignment, you should

1 Understand some of the mechanisms of the immune system.

2 Know the fundamentals of simple tests for allergies.

3 Know the degrees of addiction and how they relate to your health.

4 Know the levels of allergic reactions and how they apply to you.

The Immune System

Before you continue with Class Four, review your answers to Dr. Randolph's Chemical Questionnaire. Your answers will be very helpful in determining your treatment. A large measure of the treatment is the avoidance of chemical irritants. The severity of your illness will perhaps influence the degree of avoidance.

To help you have a better understanding of the importance of changing the conditions of your environment, we are including in its entirety a paper by Dr. Alan Levin entitled "The Hypothesis of the Immune System Dysregulation in Food and Chemical Sensitivities." The information found in this paper will be a good incentive for you to make a concerted effort to clean up your home environment.

"THE HYPOTHESIS OF IMMUNE SYSTEM DYSREGULATION IN FOOD AND CHEMICAL SENSITIVITIES"

Chemical sensitivity is an illness involving intolerance of certain chemicals found in the everyday environment. It is often referred to as a new type of allergy, and is popularly known by a variety of names: environmental illness, ecologic illness, immunotoxic syndrome, total allergy syndrome, cerebral allergy, or bioecologic illness. Doctors who treat this disorder practice Evironmental Medicine, Clinical Ecology, Ecologic Medicine, or Bioecologic Medicine.

Many physicians argue that chemical sensitivities are not an allergy at all because reactions are not mediated by the same system that causes traditional allergic reactions to pollens, dust, animal dander, and molds. Technically they are correct; we now know that chemical sensitivities are the result of a different malfunction of the immune system, recognized as a new and distinct disorder known as "immune system dysregulation."

The traditional concept of allergy associates only a few specific symptoms with a limited number of natural inhalants. In immune system dysregulation, the immune system similarly loses its ability to suppress unnecessary reactions, yet a much wider range of complex symptoms results, involving a variety of organ systems. Furthermore, these responses occur to a greater number of substances, including certain toxic chemicals as well as foods and natural inhalants. The most extreme manifestation of immune system dysregulation is universal reactivity to everything in the external environment, and even to the body's own tissues and organs.

A substance can provoke any one or more of a number of symptoms in an individual, including traditional "allergic" nasal stuffiness, wheezing, sneezing, asthma, chronic sore throat, postnasal drip, laryngitis, itching eyes, hives, and rashes. In addition, gastrointestinal disturbances such as gastric irritation, bloating, intermittent constipation or diarrhea, hemorrhoids, or anal bleeding may occur. Musculoskeletal aches, pains, or twitching, and arthritis or rheumatism are some other common reactions, as well as problems in a host of other body systems, such as frequent or painful urination, menstrual cramps, body or breath odors, metallic aftertaste, sensitivity to light, visual disturbances, and ringing in the ears.

The most surprising and dramatic documented environmentally induced symptoms by far are the cerebral and behavioral reactions. These include migraine headaches, fatigue, dizziness, learning disabilities, confusion, inability to concentrate, lack of motivation, memory loss, and dyslexia. Personality changes, mood swings, hyperactivity, and depression are also common.

In addition, another common behavioral symptom is insatiable hunger, leading to incessant eating and often to obesity. Addictions to specific foods, such as wheat, corn, sugar, coffee, and chocolate can also develop, as well as addictions to alcoholic beverages, drugs, tobacco, and even some common chemical vapors, such as perfume, hairspray, or glue.

The same immune system dysregulation which causes chemical sensitivities is also believed by some scientists to be the predecessor for such diseases as hypertension, rheumatoid arthritis, coronary artery disease, and cancer. Immune system dysregulation may also be directly responsible for certain symptoms associated with other diseases such as infectious hepatitis, herpes, and infectious mononucleosis. In addition, immune system dysregulation reduces the immune system's ability to fight infection, leaving the body vulnerable to various illnesses caused by bacteria, viruses, and fungi.

Immune system dysregulation can develop over a long period of time due to repeated infectious diseases, continuous stress, and/or cumulative exposure to toxic chemicals, even at the low levels found in our everyday environment. It can also be triggered by a single serious viral infection, major stress, or massive chemical exposure.

Immune system dysregulation often remains undiagnosed, however, because many physicians, faced with its incredible array of seemingly unrelated symptoms, and unfamiliar with the available diagnostic methods, misdiagnose it as "stress," "psychosomatic disease," or the like. The medications commonly prescribed for these problems may suppress the symptoms to some extent but often further aggravate the problems without dealing with the underlying disease process at all.

It is important to comprehend how the immune system works in order to understand how a simple malfunction can lead to such complex reactivity and symptomatology. The immune system is the body's basic defense against disease, providing protection by recognizing dangerous bacteria or viruses which enter the body and rendering them harmless. It works mainly through three kinds of white blood cells: *B-cells* from the bone marrow, *T-cells* from the thymus, and *macrophages* from the bone marrow and spleen.

B-cells produce *antibodies*, proteins which circulate in the bloodstream, locating and identifying foreign substances, which are called *antigens*. When an antigen enters the body, B-cells spring into action and produce specific antibodies which attach to the antigens to form *immune complexes*. B-cells are capable of producing a broad range of specific antibodies which identify and bind not only to disease-producing viruses and fungi, but to non-disease–producing antigens as well. B-cells are always ready to respond to foreign substances: left to function on their own, they would continuously and indiscriminately produce antibodies to all antigens, whether harmless or dangerous.

T-cells control the B-cells. When a harmless substance enters the body, the T-cells signal the B-cells to suppress antibody production; yet when a dangerous substance enters and must be eliminated, the T-cells allow antibody production, at a controlled rate and only until no more are needed. T-cells can be programmed through vaccination or immunization to allow antibody production to previously unfamiliar but harmful antigens such as smallpox or polio. Conversely, allergy shots or other immunostimulation techniques can program T-cells to recognize harmless antigens and to suppress production of their antibodies.

The macrophages filter the immune complexes (formed by the combination of foreign antigens with antibodies from the B-cells) from the blood and digest them into their component parts: proteins, carbohydrates, and lipids. These components can then be either utilized as nutrients or eliminated through the kidneys or gastrointestinal tract. The inherent capacity of the macrophage system for processing immune complexes varies among different individuals and is determined by heredity.

When a harmful antigen, such as a flu virus, enters the body, the T-cells allow the B-cells to produce flu virus antibodies and attach them to the flu virus antigens. After the resulting immune complexes have been filtered out and digested by the macrophages, the body has been effectively protected. When a substance such as wheat enters, which the body does not need to be protected from, the T-cells prevent the B-cells from producing wheat antibodies.

This same immune system mechanism which protects the body from disease can, when malfunctioning, cause a broad range of symptoms in reaction to a number of harmless or even beneficial substances entering the body. This malfunction commonly originates when the T-cells are damaged by toxic chemicals, stress, and/or infectious disease. When the normal complement of T-cells is reduced in number, or when their ability to function is impaired, they can no longer adequately control B-cell production of antibodies. Without this control, the B-cells cannot distinguish harmless dust, pollen, animal hair, or vital and nutritious foods from toxic chemicals or life-threatening bacteria or viruses. They react by producing antibodies to all foreign substances indiscriminately at an uncontrolled rate. Sometimes even *autoantibodies*—antibodies directed against the body's own tissues—are produced. Unlimited antibody production leads to the formation of larger quantities of immune complexes than the macrophages can process. When the macrophages become overloaded, the excess immune complexes are discharged into the blood-stream. These circulating complexes can then cause symptoms in any part of the body fed by an artery or capillary.

This disease process can be effectively reversed by protecting the T-cells from stressful factors, allowing them to regenerate naturally and resume their normal regulatory function. The most effective way to accomplish this is a comprehensive reduction of all possible stresses on the immune system, both physiological and psychological. Approaches to consider include the following:

ATTITUDE Develop a positive, productive attitude towards life; cultivate a sense of responsibility and purpose, and seek socially effective activities and interaction.

STRESS   Develop proper stress-management techniques, and make life changes necessary to reduce unwanted stress.

CHEMICALS   Minimize exposure to toxic chemicals in air, foods, and water. Live, eat, and work in the cleanest environment possible. Avoid cigarette smoke particularly.

EXERCISE   Include a program of regular exercise.

LIGHT   Insure adequate exposure to the benefits of natural or full-spectrum light. Conventional fluorescent lights are a stress for many with chemical sensitivities.

HARMFUL DISEASE AGENTS   Exposure to infectious bacteria, viruses, and fungi (particularly Candida albicans) should be avoided. Effective treatment should be instituted for any existing disorders from these agents. If you must be treated with antibiotics, be sure to ask your doctor for an antifungal medicine as well, to maintain proper balance among intestinal flora. Have gamma globulin injections if you have been exposed to mononucleosis or hepatitis. Avoid herpes infections.

FOOD AND NUTRITION   Obtain proper nutrition and avoid chemical contaminants by eating a balanced diet of whole, naturally produced foods. Avoid those foods that cause reactions, and rotate foods to avoid development of new sensitivities. Use nutritional supplements if individual needs exceed nutrients available from tolerated foods. Remember that individuals with immune system problems often require more of particular nutrients than the norm.

IMMUNOSTIMULATION TECHNIQUES   These include specific antigen therapy (allergy shots) or nonspecific immunological enhancement using Transfer factor, Interferon, or Thymosin. The actual healing process from immune system dysregulation is long, slow, and punctuated by exasperating short-term setbacks. These setbacks are inevitable, as the healing process invariably follows a "roller coaster" pattern. The frequency, duration, and severity of setbacks gradually diminishes until symptoms are mild and occur only occasionally.

After recovery has begun, an individual will often begin to notice adverse reactions to substances that previously caused no problems, such as diesel fumes, air pollution, or fabric finishes. This phenomenon, known as "unmasking", occurs when the elimination of dominant exposures allows underlying sensitivities to become temporarily more acute. This is to be expected. Though it is sometimes perceived as an increase of symptoms or severity of the disease, it is, in fact, an indication of improvement.

Another aspect of the healing process is the experience of withdrawal from previously unrecognized addictions. As in any traditional addiction, the feeling of well-being is maintained only through continual re-exposure to the addicting agent. Upon avoidance, this feeling of well-being gives way to various symptoms, some of which may be rather severe. This withdrawal may be experienced from a remarkably wide variety of substances, including coffee, tobacco, alcoholic beverages, many foods, and even some common chemicals. It is not uncommon, for instance, to find an individual who is "addicted to his work"; the painter who "feels miserable" on weekends; or the printer who stays drunk all during his vacation. Generally, however, withdrawal symptoms last for only three to five days and then, if the individual can avoid succumbing to temptation, the symptoms are relieved. After having abstained for long periods, a formerly addicted individual will usually have immediate and severe symptoms upon re-exposure to the addicting agent, whether it be paint, cigarettes, or wheat.

Rebuilding the immune system and regaining tolerance to chemicals and other substances in the environment is a gradual process that may take one or two years. During this time, avoidance of disease-causing agents and stress is crucial, but perhaps the most important requisite for recovery is avoidance of the toxic chemicals found in the everyday environment.

Even the elimination of a single significant chemical exposure (e.g., gas heat, smoking, or perfume) may immediately reduce symptoms and allow the healing process to begin, but it is the continuous protection of the immune system from chemical exposures of all kinds that will allow tolerance and health to be regained. Remember, however, that once the immune system has been damaged, it will always remain vulnerable. Regardless of the level of tolerance achieved, chemically-sensitive individuals should continue to minimize chemical exposures throughout their lives.

Once health is restored, occasional chemical exposures can be tolerated, giving an overall nontoxic lifestyle. The proper balance must be maintained between these greater exposures and a generally low baseline level of exposure, so that the immune system is not overloaded to the point of malfunctioning. For instance, if you must live in the city and work in a toxic, poorly ventilated office environment, you should spend as many breaks and lunch periods as possible away from smoke-filled coffee rooms and outside in clean air—in a park, on a roof garden, anywhere where you can breathe fresh outdoor air. You should also live in as clean a house and location as possible, and leave the city for unpolluted air whenever you can. If you suffer a major exposure, such as being trapped behind a diesel truck in a traffic jam for an extended period, you may require several hours at the beach breathing clean air.

It is very likely that many individuals are needlessly suffering from immune system dysregulation, without knowing about the disease or its symptoms. Because anyone is susceptible to this illness, it is beneficial for everyone to minimize exposure to toxic chemicals.

Doing Your Own Testing

(Before doing any testing, complete the entire assignment for Class Four.)

With the cost of medical services rising, people are of necessity trying to reduce medical bills. The least expensive way, of course, is prevention. To practice prevention properly, you must cut down on the things that are known to make people ill. Even more important, you must eliminate those things that are *now* affecting your state of health. For the latter, you must do testing. Many tests you can do at home if you are only mildly allergic and if you are in general good health.

Before doing any testing, you should have a thorough physical to rule out any organic medical problem other than allergy. Don't take any chances, especially if you have some chronic illness. Consult a physician knowledgeable in the field of environmental illness, so that he and his staff can supervise any testing you do at home while you are waiting for an appointment.

WARNING: *Never fast for more than one day without the close supervision of a doctor.* The purpose of fasting is to withdraw from the foods and chemicals in your body. This withdrawal can be as severe and dangerous as withdrawal from hard drugs. Some people fast for one day for religious reasons, but those people who experience headaches, dizziness, and other discomforts are probably allergic and are undergoing the beginnings of withdrawal.

Your Temperature and Pulse

Before attempting any type of testing, it would be wise for you to check your pulse and temperature each morning for a week. If these are approximately the same each morning, you can use them as a barometer in your testing. Check your temperature five minutes before and twenty minutes after each test. A change in temperature sometimes indicates a reaction. As for your pulse, check it five minutes before and twenty, forty, and sixty minutes after each test. If there is an increase or decrease of ten or more counts per minute, it is usually indicative of a reaction.

When taking your pulse for testing, the common practice of counting your pulse for fifteen seconds and multiplying it by four will not work. When doing testing, you must take your pulse for a full sixty seconds, because it can speed up or slow down intermittently.

To take your pulse on your left wrist, use the balls of the two fingers next to your right thumb. Place the fingers on the left side of the inside of the wrist about one inch above the hand. When you feel a throbbing, you have located the pulse. You can also take your pulse by placing the balls of the same two fingers on the side of your neck under your jawbone, about halfway between the chin and the ear.

Keep a diary of your pulse and temperature changes. Your records can be a big help to your doctor and can cut down the cost of professional tests.

Physical Changes

Another way to test for reactions is to observe physical changes in your appearance, particularly in your hands and face. Before and after testing, look at the color of your skin, fingernails, and the whites of your eyes. Take note of any changes in color.

Further, you can test your coordination by samples of your handwriting. At four different times and on four different pieces of paper, write your name, address, and telephone number in pencil. It does not matter what you write as long as the same thing is written on each of the four pieces of paper. Write it once before the test, and then again five minutes, thirty minutes, and six hours after the test. Be sure to label each sample. Don't compare any of the papers until you have completed the fourth one. A deterioration in the quality of your penmanship after the test indicates that the tested material affects your coordination.

It is always helpful to have someone else observe you during your testing. Besides observing all of the things you do, your observer may notice things that would escape you, such as restless legs, scratching yourself, irritability, or some other behavioral changes.

Time Between Tests

There are harmless ways to test yourself for reactions to foods, chemicals in foods, and chemicals in the air.

Always wait three days between tests. If you have delayed reactions and your tests are spaced too close to each other, you won't be able to detect the excitant, i.e., the irritant that causes your problem. If you are unsure about what the test showed, wait a week without testing anything else and try testing that one item again.

Food Testing

Before you do any food testing, it is important that you read Chapters 8 and 9 in *Coping With Your Allergies*, to become familiar with related foods.

Henry T., a man in his twenties, mentioned to Jeannie, a knowledgeable friend, that he was having trouble clearing up an acne condition. He had been to several doctors, including a dermatologist. Medications had only aggravated the condition. Jeanne asked Henry a few questions about his diet and suggested that Henry avoid eating cheese and any food containing milk. Within a few days his face showed improvement and cleared up by the end of the month.

Henry's problem with acne was a very simple case, but it does illustrate the point that food allergy can be caused by eating a food too frequently. That was the clue that Jeanne used to suggest avoiding cheese and milk products. She found that Henry ate cheese every day, frequently more than once a day.

If Jeanne had been a professional, she would have known that when you avoid milk, you should also avoid beef because cow's milk and beef are related foods.

There are four circumstances under which you should suspect a particular food:

1 When you eat it every day.

2 When you crave it.

3 When you have been feeling discomfort and eating a particular food makes you feel better.

4 When you feel a discomfort, such as a cough, a headache, or another symptom, right after eating a particular food.

If you are planning to test a food, you must avoid the food for a specific period of time. If you do not do this, the test will not be valid. It must be long enough to unmask the symptoms but not so long that you can readapt to the food. The average time for unmasking is four days. People have been known to readapt within twelve days. The test, therefore, will be valid if you avoid the food for five to eleven days. To play it safe, we suggest you avoid the food for a period of seven to ten days.

After the proper period of avoidance, eat half a cup or a few tablespoons of the food before eating anything else that day. Wait for an hour. If symptoms occur immediately, you probably have an allergy to that food. If there is no immediate reaction or if the reaction is minor, and you wish to confirm it, eat or drink as much of that food as you can during that day. This type of test will not prove that you are *not* allergic to the food. If, however, you have a change in behavior or other health problems within eighteen hours after you've stopped eating the food, you can be quite sure that this is an allergy. If the test is not conclusive, it may be because other unknown allergies are muddying up the picture.

If you are allergic to a food, avoid it and, if possible, other related foods for three to six months. You may find that you can regain a tolerance for it. Once you've regained your tolerance, eat the food only once a week, or, at most, once every fifth day, so you won't reactivate your allergy.

Food Additive Testing

Larry W., a normally healthy medical student, became curious about all that was being written concerning additives in foods. He convinced his roommates, Ed and Jack, to experiment with him. For three weeks they changed their diets to avoid eating foods with artificial color, artificial flavor, and preservatives. This was the only change that they made. Jack discovered that he had much more energy. Bob, however, was the one who was the most surprised. Since childhood, he had experienced an irregular heartbeat that had always concerned him. As a result of this experiment, Bob found that his heartbeat was regular as long as he avoided artificial additives in his food.

If you wish to discover the effects of additives on your own health, the best way to do so is to do your own cooking from scratch for a period of three weeks. Make sure that you use no additives, no foods containing additives (you will have to read labels very carefully), and no prepackaged foods. You will note that the avoidance period for food additives is longer than for food testing. It appears that it sometimes takes longer for the body to clear itself of chemicals.

We do not intend to give the impression that the food additive test just mentioned was a *conclusive* test. There are ways that this test could be misleading. Health problems that persist even during the test could indicate that there are additional factors causing the problem, and the removal of one excitant (irritant) may not be enough to show a marked improvement.

Even a minor improvement in behavior or well-being indicates that one should pursue testing, and would be wise to take preventive measures seriously. It is important enough to repeat here that any condition can be something other than allergy and *must be checked by a physician.*

Simple Tests for Airborne Chemicals

There are two ways of conducting simple chemical tests. The first one is used if you suspect a particular product but aren't sure. In this case, you avoid the chemical for two or three weeks and then test it.

Jane C. suddenly developed headaches that were particularly bad in the morning when she awakened. She drew up a chart that contained the following information:

- Approximate date of the onset of the headache
- Any new purchases around that time
- Any new procedures or activities starting at that time
- Time and place where the headache began
- Time and place where the headache seemed worse

As a result of this chart, she began to suspect her new digital wristwatch that she never removed. She stopped wearing the watch and the headaches stopped. To check out her findings and her conclusion, she wore it one night and the headache returned. Her headaches had been worse in the morning because she had always slept on her side with her hand supporting her head. In her case, it turned out to be the digital watch itself, but it could have been only the plastic watch band. Jane's procedure to self-test for the cause of her headache is recommended. Of course, the cause may not be as readily detected, but the procedure is worth noting.

The second simple chemical test involves putting a sample of the product in a tightly sealed jar. Leave it in the jar for at least forty-eight hours or until you are ready to take the test. This type of test should be done when the air quality outdoors is in the "good" range. First, go for a long brisk walk. As soon as you return, open the jar and hold the product under your nose for thirty minutes, unless you notice an immediate change in how you feel or look. If there is no change but you still suspect the chemical, close the jar until bedtime. Then open it again, placing it as close to your bed as possible. If it is a soft product, such as a fabric, put it on your pillow and sleep on it.

There are other ways to test for minor sensitivities to specific chemicals. For example, you may suspect tap water because you don't enjoy drinking it, because it tastes funny, or because you don't feel well when you drink it in large quantities. Or, you may want to test it simply because the public is learning that not all tap water is as good for us as we were led to believe.

To test your tap water, first find a pure water that you can drink for a week. It can be a pure well water, spring water, or distilled water. It must be bottled in glass, otherwise the test may indicate a sensitivity to plastic. For best results with this test, all foods that you eat should be washed (or at least rinsed) and cooked in the pure water.

On the eighth day, drink a half-gallon of *tap* water, unless you begin to react more quickly. Any symptoms experienced at this time could indicate a sensitivity to the tap water.

For other tests, refer to the basic books for this course: *Coping With Your Allergies* and *Allergies and the Hyperactive Child.* Additional tests will be found in *The Type 1/Type 2 Allergy Relief Program.*

If you are at home, taking this course under the supervision of a doctor, turn to Part III, Class Four lesson plan for further guidance. If you still have questions, consult with the physician's staff member who is supervising your education.

I. Read Class Five and be prepared to discuss it.

As you read the assigned portions of *Coping With Your Allergies*, you will see that it details the toxins found in your home. Wherever possible, safer alternatives are suggested. As you prepare a list of the changes you wish to make in your environment both now and in the future, bear in mind that toxins are poisons that stress even the healthy immune system. Naturally, the more quickly you clean up your home environment, the easier it will be to strengthen your immune system. However, "Don't try to be a 100 percenter!" it is important to understand the whole picture so that you can make your own choices.

II. Complete the assigned readings and answer all questions.

  A. *Coping with Your Allergies*

    1. Chapter 17, P pages 169–178 or H pages 155–163.

      a. What can you substitute for oil-sprayed or hexachlorophene-treated filters in heating and cooling equipment?

      b. If the odor of turpentine bothers you, what related substances should you avoid?

    2. Chapter 18, P pages 179–183 or H pages 164–167.

      a. List the first three steps to take to eliminate problems in your home.

      b. Without trying to be a 100 percenter, list the steps you could take to clean up your bedroom, clothing, and food.

    3. Chapter 19, P pages 184–192 or H pages 168–175.

      a. List plastic products that you use at home or work that could be replaced with more ecological products.

      b. Read each of the miscellaneous tips. Note which can be put into effect immediately without additional expense.

    4. Chapter 20, P pages 193–196 or H pages 176–178.

Explain how the telephone not only saves you gasoline, but adds to your health.

5. Chapter 21, P pages 197–202 or H pages 179–183.

   a. How can you order medic alert?

   b. To make up an ecological first-aid kit, what products can you find in your home?

6. Chapter 22, P pages 203–208 or H pages 184–189.

   a. What is Dr. Rinkel's axiom for doctors and how does it benefit you?

   b. If your doctor is not a clinical ecologist, how can you introduce multiple chemical sensitivities to him so that he will take you seriously?

7. Chapter 26, P pages 256–273 or H pages 229–246.

   a. Find something made of inexpensive, white, untreated cotton. Use the water bubble test to check that it is untreated. Place it on a table with some permanent-press cotton and some polyester. Use the "crawly feeling" test to see if you can feel the difference.

   b. Name three other ways to test fabrics.

8. Chapter 27, P pages 274–280 or H pages 247–253. Make a list of your home furnishings that will need to be replaced in the near future. State briefly how the information in this chapter may influence your purchases.

9. Chapter 28, P pages 281–288 or H pages 254–260. Select inexpensive, nontoxic cosmetic preparations. Compare the cost with your current products to see how much money you can save as you practice prevention.

10. Chapter 30, P pages 301–306 or H pages 272–276.

B. From the *Yeast Connection:*

   1. Read pages vii to xii. In the paperback edition, vii-xii are the unnumbered pages that follow "A Special Message for the Physician" and precede the Table of Contents. Read P pages 2-55 or H pages 2-53.

   2. Read "Yeast Revisited," Textbook Class Five and complete the exercises as directed.

Class Five

PREVIEW

Detecting the causes of complex allergies is not simple, but it can be accomplished. Systematic procedures must be followed faithfully, but all answers may be available only after weeks or months of testing. The entire environment should be examined as far as it is in your control to do so. Once you know the offending allergens, you can embark on a program for a toxic-free life. Again, this will take time to do thoroughly and it will incur some expense and some change in life habits. Happily, the good results of toxic-free living are a great comfort to the extremely sensitive and a valuable assurance to the moderately allergic patient. The improvement can be faster if you practice good breathing exercises daily.

The role of yeast in our lives is of particular concern because of the culture and food habits of Americans and because of the practices of the American food industry. Daily exposures to allergens must be expected because of limits to one's controls over the environment. You *can* learn to live with these exposures.

OBJECTIVES

After studying Class Five and its assignment, you should be able to:

1 Understand the concept of Management of Complex Allergies.

2 Set up procedures to detect allergy problems.

3 Begin a relatively toxic-free life.

4 Understand the nature of a yeast problem and how to discuss it with your doctor.

5 Know methods to help you function while exposed to irritants.

Complex Allergies

Detecting the Problems

As you read the boldface headings in Chapter 17 of *Coping With Your Allergies* (Drugs and Medications, Pesticides, etc.), make note of these categories of substances in your own environment. A look in your medicine cabinet and on your bathroom shelves will alert you to non-drug items that you may otherwise overlook—after-shave lotion, depilatory creams, and even your shower cap or shower curtain. A look under the sink may reveal powders, liquids, and cleaning pads that you may have forgotten about. And so, too, might a systematic examination of other rooms in the house reveal unsuspected irritants.

The Toxic-Free Life

Perhaps the greatest benefit you can get from reading Chapter 18 of *Coping With Your Allergies* will be the encouragement that your effort will pay off in better health. Some results may be immediate; others may not even be noticeable for some time. Be patient; you will improve.

In Appendix E of *Allergies and the Hyperactive Child*, the authors state that "... allergies can be caused by various items within your home. In a few hours or days, symptoms can be entirely relieved after making a few changes." The rewards are many and can be lasting—so long as the commitment is lasting.

Breathing

In *Coping With Your Allergies*, the authors state that "the key to relaxation and stress reduction is giving up control of your breathing. It is extremely difficult to control your breathing if, as you exhale, you drop your jaw and shoulders, think 'Relax,' and let your body go limp."

Although the section on breathing exercises was previously assigned, it bears repeating at this point:

In the beginning you will practice these exercises lying down. Later you will learn to incorporate them into your daily life so that you may practice them standing, sitting, or walking around.

Relaxation Breathing. Place one hand on your diaphragm and the other on your lower abdomen. As you breathe in, force your lower abdomen to swell like a balloon. As you slowly breathe out, drop your jaw and shoulders. Try to imagine oxygen passing through each part of your body as you think, "I am relaxing my jaw, shoulders, arms, chest, hips, legs, feet." Let each part go limp as you think of it.

Count Breathing (to increase lung capacity). Inhale totally, filling your lungs by the count of four; hold to the count of four; exhale, emptying your lungs by the count of four. Repeat several times. Increase the count, gradually moving up to a count of six, then eight, etc. But do not increase it to a point of strain.

Chest Breathing Interlock your fingers and press them against your chest as you breathe out, emptying your lungs. Retain the pressure so that on your next breath your lungs must work harder. Press again against your chest as you breathe out. Relax and allow a full breath, then repeat.

Breathing Breaks. To relax, try to do five repeats of relaxation breathing exercise, at least every hour.

Keep these breathing exercises, as well as the stress reduction program, in mind as you read the next section.

Coping with Unavoidable Daily Exposures

When you are extremely sensitive (i.e., when your immune system has broken down), there are limits as to the amount of chemical exposure your body can safely handle. Nevertheless, unless you spend all of your time in a specially-created "clean" environment, you are going to come in contact with environmental allergens—at work, at school, in stores, and elsewhere. You will also contact them while traveling to and from any location. Whatever the degree of your sensitivities, it is important to take precautions so that you do not overload your body with toxins and allergens.

The concept of overloading is central to all of the suggestions presented here. If, for example, ten substances are particularly harmful to you and you encounter all ten simultaneously, you are likely to be very uncomfortable because you have overloaded your system. If, on the other hand, you have been able to limit your exposure to only two, you are going to have less of a problem. The following suggestions are aimed at minimizing harmful exposures so that, as much as possible, you can maintain your normal daily activities.

Before You Go Out

Before leaving your home, be sure to allow yourself at least twenty minutes to do whatever relaxation techniques work best for you (see Chapter 7, "Stress Reduction" in *Coping With Your Allergies*. It is important to leave home in as relaxed a state as possible. The breathing exercises we have discussed in this class could be a very good beginning.

While You Are Out

It is important to condition yourself so that, while you are being exposed (as you drive a car or move about), you can maintain the relaxed state in which you left home. If you are relaxed, your body can tolerate more chemical stress. Whether or not you feel physically or emotionally stressed, you should take five minutes every hour to establish a relaxation pattern by doing some breathing exercises and by drinking at least one glass of good, pure spring water.

Often while driving a car, you will be chemically exposed. You may pass an area where workmen are repairing a road with tar, you may find yourself caught in a traffic jam, or you may be temporarily stuck behind a truck or bus from which exhaust is blowing right at you. While being exposed, avoid deep breathing to minimize exposure. As soon as you have passed the bad area, open the car window, take a deep breath, and then exhale noisily, clearing your lungs. Follow this by doing some deep-breathing exercises.

If you have a confrontation with someone, deep breathing when you are clear of the stressful situation will help. Both interpersonal confrontations and chemical exposures are stresses on your system, and it is imperative to minimize the detrimental effects of both. Proper breathing exercises relax you in these difficult periods.

When You Return Home

After any experience away from your home, which is now relatively toxic-free, you have been exposed to many irritants. You have been exposed to all kinds of fumes; they are on your clothes, on your body, and in your hair. To dispose of these contaminants as quickly as possible, follow these instructions:

1   Go to a part of the house that you do not regularly use, such as the basement or a storeroom. Remove your clothes. Do not take these clothes into your bedroom, bathroom, or kitchen. These are the three areas in which you spend the most time while you are at home. Go to your bathroom, shower, wash your hair, and come out wearing clean clothes. In this way, you will rid yourself of the allergens you encountered outside your home.

2   After you have cleansed yourself, if you are on oxygen, it is a good idea at this point to take the oxygen for six minutes. One hour later, take it for another six minutes.

3   It is not a good idea to begin eating as soon as you come home. Give your system an opportunity to get rid of some of the toxins first. One way to do this is to drink several glasses of pure spring water. If you do not feel well, another way is to take alkali salts, milk of magnesia, vitamin C, or whatever you use to clear your system when you are having a bad reaction. The object is to cleanse your system without waiting until your symptoms develop into a *severe* reaction. Still another way of ridding your body of any accumulated toxins is to do the various exercises you use to keep in shape.

4   After exposure it is particularly unwise to eat any food that has given you trouble in the past. It is also a bad time to combine foods or to test foods.

When a person finds out that he has many sensitivities, the tendency is to retreat from the world to a totally "safe" and predictable place. Sometimes that is necessary, for a while. But retreat can be both psychologically and physically disastrous if overdone. The aim of clinical ecology is not to make people outcasts, but to teach them how to cope with our polluted 20th century world. You should begin to go out into the world as soon as you are able. It is very important that you maintain the proper perspective, the proper positive "mental attitude" (see Chapter 30, "Mental Attitude," in *Coping With Your Allergies*).

The techniques described here are all useful even for the person who is 100 percent healthy. These practices should not be considered as a chore that must be done just because you are "sick" or "allergic," but rather as exercises designed to build up your body so that you can get the most out of life.

When dealing with a suppressed immune system, it is essential to remember that such a system can tolerate very little stress. Thus, you want to make sure to avoid an overload. When you must be exposed to environmental stress, reduce the emotional stress and the food stress. It is a matter of balancing your exposures so that you can maintain an optimum level of good health.

Yeast Revisited

By now you have probably heard that many environmentally ill patients have serious health problems related to yeast. That is why, in a previous class, you learned the names of foods that contain yeast and molds. As you read the assigned pages in *The Yeast Connection*, it is important for you to notice the similarities between symptoms of food and chemical sensitivities and those of Candida. *Be very careful not to make snap judgments about your health as a result of this information.* Susceptibility in this case is not something you can judge by yourself. Read the material, and if you suspect you have a problem related to Candida, it is important that you discuss the matter with your doctor.

Read H page x or P unnumbered page that follows "A Special Message for the Physician." It is entitled "Are Your Health Problems Yeast Connected?" Answer the ten questions. This will give you some indication of whether or not yeast "possibly" plays a role in your symptoms. At the risk of being repetitious, notice that the yeast connection is only one possibility. In no way does it suggest that it is the total problem.

Read pages 17–28. Make a list of any symptoms and practices related to your problems.

Fill out the "Candida Questionnaire and Score Sheet" on pages 29–33. Total up your score to help you have a clear picture of the possible yeast connection. Take note that every one of the major symptoms in Section B on pages 31–32, and Section C on pages 32–33 are also found in the lists of symptoms that can be caused by food and the environment.

If you are at home, taking this course under the supervision of a doctor, turn to Part III, Class Five lesson plan for further guidance. If you still have questions, consult with the physician's staff member who is supervising your education.

ASSIGNMENT FOR CLASS SIX

I. Read Class Six and be prepared to discuss it.
  A. List unquestioned answers about adaptation.
  B. List additional constructive ideas you have have about gaining cooperation from family and from a support group.

II. Complete the assigned readings and answer all questions about them. Assigned readings for Class Six are from *The Type 1/Type 2 Allergy Relief Program.*
  A. Chapter 1, P pages 1–24 or H pages 13–36.
    1. Read the symptoms of a Type 1 and a Type 2.
    2. By taking the test on P pages 21–24 or H pages 32–35, decide if you are a Type 1, a Type 2, a combination of both, or neither.
    3. Note the check list on P pages 17–20 or H pages 29–36, particularly the part of the list detailing what allergy is *not*. See if you have any symptoms. Consult your doctor if in doubt.
  B. Chapter 2, P pages 25–51 or H pages 37–62.
    1. For Type 1, name three office tests, two lab tests, and two home tests. Compare the home tests with those detailed in the section entitled "Doing Your Own Testing" in Class Four.
    2. What severe symptoms should warn you against home testing?
  C. Chapter 3, P pages 53–84 or H pages 63–93.
    1. Name home, lab and office tests for Type 2.
    2. How do the home tests agree with the section entitled, "Doing You Own Testing"?

III. Review.
  A. Check back over the classes. If you have questions for which you have found no answers, bring them to the last session.
  B. If any of your questions relates specifically to your own health problem, make an appointment for a private consultation.

Class Six

PREVIEW

All of us can reduce our reactions to various substances, especially by avoiding them. But once we have given our bodies a chance to recover, we can rebuild our adaptation potential. A number of healthy practices have been recommended in this course, and all of them should be kept in mind and followed during this period of rebuilding. How much or how far the rebuilding can go is a highly individual matter. You do not live in a vacuum nor on an isolated island. It is important for you to know how to deal with your family, and learn how to deal with your susceptibility.

OBJECTIVES

After studying Class Six and its assignment, you should be able to

1 Recognize many symptoms that are not allergy.

2 Follow the steps in rebuilding your adaptation.

3 Use and recommend to others the various support groups for environmentally-ill people.

Type 1/Type 2 Reading

Because symptoms of environmental illness are the ones most frequently overlooked by the average physician, they were given priority in the first Classes of this course.

In *Allergies and the Hyperactive Child, An Alternative Approach to Allergies*, and *Coping With Your Allergies*, you have already covered chapters that teach you how to recognize your symptoms. You have read, also, how to determine if you have chemical susceptibilities and even how to test yourself.

You may question, then, why you should read about symptoms and tests in *The Type 1/Type 2 Allergy Relief Program*. Frankly, this material is more than repetition. The book is included in the course because it helps to give you a new perspective on your symptoms. In the preface we told you that "the main goal . . . is to wean the patient away from the doctor and to teach the patient to be more self-sufficient."

While you are being tested and doing some of your own testing under supervision, your doctor will recognize any symptoms unrelated to environmental illness. When you begin to wean yourself from your doctor, the information in *The Type 1/Type 2 Allergy Relief Program* will help you recognize the difference between symptoms that are allergy related and those that are not.

Rebuilding Adaptation

Adaptation is the ability of the body to maintain its homeostasis—the body's balance. The way in which the temperature of the body changes under different conditions is a good example of homeostasis. When the storekeeper goes into a frozen-food locker, his body temperature changes as the body heats itself. On a hot day, one's body temperature is reduced as the body cools itself. As long as the body can adapt to the temperature of the environment, it remains on an even keel.

When the body comes in contact with other factors of the environment it reacts to adapt itself to the new, strange conditions. As long as these changes take place in a reasonable period of time between stimulus and effect, the body stays healthy. But when there is a decrease in adaptation, ecologic illness results.

After you have learned to reduce your reactions and have given your body a chance to recover, it is important to rebuild your adaptation. To help you understand this process we have included a report about a group of patients who were helped by Dr. James Carroll Cox of suburban Washington, D.C. The patients participating in his project were extremely sensitive and without much hope of functioning again in the "normal world."

The procedures described in this report are recommended only as a guide to help you after you have stabilized your diet and improved your environment. Before you decide the extent of your involvement in a readaptive program, consider three things: the degree of your illness, the number of foods and chemicals that cause reactions, and your own timetable. Usually, you can make the best judgments about the timetable. Of course you should consult with your doctor or counselor when you have *any* doubts about proceeding.

"REBUILDING ADAPTATION, A REPORT"

Regaining Foods

Since the patients had already received their initial testing, they were placed on a rotary diet, eating one food per meal, two or three meals a day, on a four-, five-, or seven-day cycle, according to the degree of sensitivity. When possible, these included only safe foods, even if the foods had to be exotic wild game and foreign foods. Universal food reactors used foods that had been tested + or –1 and, when necessary, + or –2. All other foods were avoided for a period of three to six months, depending on the degree of sensitivity.

The patients, having been taught to use relaxation techniques, were advised to use them before eating and prior to any new testing. This helped to allay their fears of testing without local supervision. First they tested foods they had never previously eaten, and then they graduated to retesting their + or –1 foods and then their + or –2s. Those who wished to retest + or –3s and + or –4s were advised to do so under medical supervision even though they had to travel great distances to do so. As reports came back that some + or –3 foods were cyclic and were again tolerated, some patients ventured to test even their + or –3s by themselves.

We found that some patients who had been doing well for a year or two would suddenly lose ground and find all their major complaints returning; they also were having new symptoms. When they were questioned, it was discovered that they had become careless with their rotation. It was concluded that even after the diet was stabilized, the safest way to keep from backsliding was to continue rotating indefinitely. Patients who did so reported that it not only maintained their health, it helped them regain a tolerance for many foods; they reported a general increase in adaptation.

Those who "cheated" did it frequently and kept losing ground. Human nature being what it is, we know that there must always be exceptions for any rule or procedure. To satisfy this need, a plan was devised to train patients to adapt to eating patterns necessary at social functions—a dinner party or a meal in a restaurant. One idea came from a practice used by some business executives. They take two tablespoons of oil before drinking at business parties. They say that this enables them to tolerate more alcohol with less effect.

Before eating an "unsafe" meal, some patients started taking two tablespoons of a food oil that was included on their rotation of that particular day. We have since learned the possible merit of this procedure. In a paper Dr. Randolph once reported that some patients could eat otherwise untolerated foods if they were stir-fried in oil. Dr. Randolph has said that he believes the stir-fry method coats the food in oil which in turn slows down the absorption rate; a major factor in food allergy is the rate of absorption. Whatever the reason, some patients reported success with the oil.

For the first few attempts in breaking their diet, some patients took further preventive measures. Immediately after the meal, even before they began to react, they took their alkaline salts or milk of magnesia. At the slightest reaction, they were taught to take a spring water enema as soon as possible. Pure vitamin C in large quantities can be an anti-allergic measure. A large quantity may cause loose stools or diarrhea in certain individuals. If this occurs, simply decrease the dose of vitamin C. (Check first with your physician).

The approach was most successful when it was deliberate and

controlled rather than haphazard food exposure. The plan was to attempt to rebuild adaptation, following the same principle of optimum dose treatment.

To reduce the stress the system had experienced, each exposure was followed by a cleansing period. This consisted of a return, for several days, to a diet of one food per meal, even though the patient had advanced to multiple food meals. Graudally they increased the amount of food and the number of meals they could tolerate for one exposure.

Each patient learned that he had to discover his own time frame. The process was so successful that some reported that they could indulge all Thanksgiving Day and be able to repeat the process by Christmas. Gradually, some extremely sensitive patients adapted well enough to travel for a week or two, eating in restaurants. They were advised to proceed as cautiously as possible, rotating when able to do so, and avoiding things like stews, fried foods, and "fast food fare." While caution was strongly advised, they were also counseled not to fret, and become agitated and tense over matters they could not control. To help reduce stress, the following were recommended: exercise, breathing exercise, consumption of great quantities of tolerated water, and the relaxation techniques taught to them by Dr. Cox.

Sometimes there were foods that these people found themselves tempted or forced to eat daily. When they returned home, they found they were again addicted to these foods. A typical case was that of a traveler who had eaten eggs and potatoes every morning for two weeks. When she returned home she had to avoid eggs and potatoes. After three months, she was able to tolerate them again on rotation. I believe her case illustrates how successfully a patient can rebuild her capacity for adaptation. With each subsequent journey, she was less troubled by the food and her period of avoidance was gradually decreased. She finally reached the stage where a twelve-day avoidance was sufficient for her to reintroduce the foods into her rotation.

There were two major obstacles which discouraged patients from an indefinite (or lifetime) commitment to rotation. They complained that it was too cumbersome to make changes; there was always the danger that there would be constant exposure to a food family because of mistakes made when incorporating minor foods, such as oils, herbs, teas, etc. Also, people said that it was impossible to arrange their rotations and still enjoy their favorite recipes.

Those complaints led to the development of the formula found in Chapter 4 of *If This Is Tuesday, It Must Be Chicken*. After practicing it a few times, it enables you to change your rotation frequently, within a matter of minutes. You can make permanent or temporary changes. Without breaking your rotation, you can cook or bake any recipe from scratch.

The Chemical Environment

The patients in the project were able to rebuild some degree of adaptation to chemicals. Greater caution, however, was needed. Testing is more complicated; environmental control, more costly and time consuming; and the control of the amount of exposure, more difficult. Because overexposure to one chemical can trigger a decrease in adaptation to all chemicals, a patient can be thrown into a domino effect and lose tolerance for all chemicals. Another important factor to consider is the interaction between chemical sensitivities and food allergies. Whenever patients found a "haven" in their environment, they reported an increased tolerance for foods. Conversely, overexposure to chemicals always retriggered their food allergies.

The patients continued their own chemical testing with procedures now found in *Coping With Your Allergies*. An earlier version of the same reference book was used to clean up their homes ecologically. At that time there was little literature available, but as new books were written the patients were encouraged to read them. A major part of the program was education.

The complaints began to roll in about lack of finances, lack of strength to make the changes, and lack of family cooperation. That's when we began to apply the motto: "Don't try to be a 100 percenter who drops the whole project because he can't do it all."

An effort was made to teach each patient to plan his own priorities. Patients were trained to use Francis Silver's method "That Crawly Feeling," found in Chapter 26 of *Coping With Your Allergies*. It is of particular importance to people who suffer from a loss of smell and don't know what makes them ill, people who are addicted to odors, and, as a matter of fact, to anyone with chemical sensitivities.

Experienced patients with an acute sense of smell were trained in the Randolph method as "noses." They made house calls to detect hidden contaminants.

Even when people were handicapped by a lack of finances, they learned how to build their "haven" and lower their total load.

The process of rebuilding adaptation began after the patient had a "haven," even if it were just one small bedroom, so the patient could have at least eight hours in a comparatively pure environment.

First the patients would have to reach a level of reasonable comfort in which they could function—call it "Plateau A." They would then take a deliberate minute exposure to some chemical and proceed in the way described for rebuilding food adaptation. In effect, they were building their tolerance to the excitant (the substance that caused the reactions).

After a few successful attempts with deliberate exposure, the patients began to complain that they were sliding back for an extended period of time. Although at first it was thought that patients had taken too much exposure too quickly, later it was seen as a pattern, two steps forward, one step back, two steps forward. After the setback, when the patients improved, they would reach Plateau B, a sustained plateau of better health than that experienced in Plateau A. Because this happened to so many patients so often, it was gradually accepted as a natural process of rebuilding adaptation.

Even when the patients experienced a fairly lengthy setback, they were not so discouraged; they knew they could look forward to reaching a higher plateau. Gradually they found they could tolerate longer periods of exposure to the particular chemical. When one woman started exposure to newsprint, she had a –2 after five minutes. It would last for two or three days. Now after an hour, she experiences a –1 for an hour or two. With smoke, indirect exposure on a smoker's clothes provoked a –2 reaction within minutes. Now, after a full day in a smoke-filled room, she has a –1 for a few hours. This is true only if, as soon as she reaches her haven, she immediately washes her clothes and hair and takes a bath.

One member of the group suffered from varying reactions of –2s and –3s as well as +2s and +3s, depending on the chemical exposures. She can now be away from her haven for two or three weeks at a time, exposed to all types of toxins, including nonorganic food. If she stays away too long, she begins to "crash." Once home again, she has withdrawal symptoms, a period of setback, and then reaches a higher plateau. As long as she doesn't do it too frequently, she finds withdrawal periods less reactive and of shorter duration.

Making Choices for Exposure

An important part of the training was learning to make choices for exposures, what to avoid and what to try to adapt to. This required individual counseling to help them decide priorities. Although each patient had to find his own way, there were certain principles that could be applied. To do so, there were two ways to approach the procedure: exposure to a specific toxin, one at a time or a combination of unavoidable toxins.

Take paint as a specific toxin. Unless the patient were an artist, it was not considered necessary to try to readapt to paint. For the artist, paint was usually one of the worst offenders and would probably be one of the most difficult to gain back. When it was possible, the artist was convinced to turn to other creative endeavors that did not require the use of paints and turpentine. If that was not successful, the artist was counseled to use the readapting procedure by first practicing with some toxin that was not so troublesome to him. In time, once he found his body beginning to respond to the process, he could then attempt to paint a few minutes at a time, out of doors in a brisk wind and using every precaution possible. Gradually, by careful planning, he could increase the amount of exposure.

Everyone eventually had to deal with those toxins that are so pervasive in our society that you can't leave your house without some combined exposure to them: smoke, perfume, gas, gasoline, etc. The best way to do this was to visit the home of a good friend or relative where there was a pleasant and understanding atmosphere. In such a home, the patient, without fear of derision and criticism, could take oxygen, leave abruptly, or could go outside for a brisk walk and return if he wished.

Patients were advised to choose occasions they really enjoyed and wished to adapt to, while also being selective about the degree of exposure they would encounter. In other words, it would be counterproductive to make his first outing in a home filled with smoke from pipes, cigars, cigarettes, and a burning fireplace, and where there were crowds of people wearing heavy perfumes and other contaminates that would overwhelm the patient.

Experience has taught patients that the most valuable lesson can be learned by comparing "choosing versus cheating": carefully planned buildup of exposure versus frequent, indiscriminate, spur-of-the-moment cheating resulting in uncontrolled exposure.

Summary

Even the conventional allergist agrees that dust shots are not a license to live in a dust-filled home. So it is with an ecology patient;

testing, avoidance, and/or treatment alone are not sufficient. If patients are to return to society, they need education with guidance of a physician in a planned program. The experience of the pilot project indicates that it would have to extend beyond what can be accomplished during office hours. Patients need help and support from each other. They can receive that support from a local chapter of HEAL, the Human Ecology Action League. The pilot project suggests that such support groups can be the instrument for helping physicians help ecology patients to a speedier and safer return to the mainstream of life.

With hindsight, we can see two ways that the project would be better if conducted today. At that time there was no local clinical ecologist to guide us, so the treatment had to be restricted to education of the patient and avoidance of excitants (offending foods, chemicals, etc.). In addition, there has been such progress in the field of environmental medicine that a knowledgeable clinical ecologist today could easily speed up the process using the many innovations that have since been discovered.

Family Cooperation

To have optimum conditions for a patient there must be family cooperation. Often the success of the treatment is directly related to the amount of support given by the family. This, however, must be a two-way street. The patient must realize he is not living in a vacuum, and the family members must accept the fact that they must make certain concessions and, above all else, give total moral support.

To know how to give the best help, family members should participate in the patient-education classes, or at least do the assigned reading. They should also take an active part in the support group.

Nadine L. Hume Paulin has written excellent pamphlets for the patients, family, and friends. These booklets will give you a better understanding of the need for cooperation, especially in dealing with the extremely sensitive patient. The pamphlets are listed in the Bibliography at the end of this book under the heading *Home Aids for Recovery from Environmental Illness: For the Patient; For the Family; For Friends.*

In the following lists, the Do's and Don'ts for patient and family are grouped in a way to suggest positive approaches to solving problems and dealing with everyday relationships.

Do's and Don'ts for the Patient

1 *Don't* make unreasonable demands on your family.
   Do set up priorities and ways you can compromise and separate them from procedures you must take to protect your health.
   Do let others know that you appreciate their cooperation.

2 *Don't* expect your family to make all the concessions.
   Do set the pace by avoiding cheating with foods that cause you depression or any other behavioral manifestations that affect your family.

3 *Don't* become a chronic complainer, constantly whining about your problems.
   Do try to maintain a positive attitude at all times.
   Do join a support group of patients with whom you can share your problems.
   Do encourage your family to join the group so they can talk with cooperative families of other patients.

4 *Don't* complain about the family's perfumed products, detergents, cosmetics, etc.
   Do offer to help family members find products compatible with your health.

5 *Don't* expect others to guess what makes you ill, and don't get angry when they cannot anticipate your special needs.
   Do make a point of politely telling others what bothers you, and be prepared to suggest alternative products or procedures.

6 *Don't* use your illness as an excuse to pamper yourself.
   Do force yourself to be as independent as possible. For example, moving about to do chores will give you something to occupy yourself and help you forget your aches and pains. The exercise of movement will improve your circulation and help you purge yourself of some of your reactions.

7 *Don't* separate yourself from your family's activities.
   Do suggest family activities in which you can participate.
   Do carefully select other family outings that will give you the least amount of exposure and the greatest enjoyment.
   Do keep your chemical and food exposure at a minimum prior to the activity so you have greater tolerance.
   Do, above all else, enjoy yourself during the function without worrying about aftereffects or complaining and spoiling everyone else's fun.

8 *Don't* complain if you become ill after you have intentionally and knowingly exposed yourself to allergens.

Do remember it was your decision, that you made the choice knowing you would have to pay the consequences.

9 *Don't* become careless when participating in family activities. In the beginning you have to be extra cautious. After you start to improve, you can be more flexible.
Do remember that exposing yourself to things you cannot tolerate has an adverse effect on your immune system, which needs time and relief from exposure in order to recover.

Do's and Don'ts for the Family

1 *Don't* prejudge the patient's condition or label the patient a hypochondriac.
Do remember the term hypochondriac has been widely used by physicians who do not understand environmental illness and who sometimes use the term when they cannot make a textbook diagnosis.
Do educate yourself along with the patient so you will understand the philosophy of the illness and how to cope with it.

2 *Don't* try to dissuade the patient or try to convince the patient to return to conventional treatments that never helped.
Do remember that most environmentally-ill patients have wasted time and money, and suffered pain and discouragement, going from "specialist" to "specialist" who did not understand the nature of the illness.
Do remember that in many cases this is the last vestige of hope.
Do remember that the patient desperately needs understanding and support.
Do remember that negative feedback from the family can be more detrimental to the patient's health than any other kind of stress.

3 *Don't* try to convince the patient to do something he believes will make him ill.
Do learn to recognize the objective symptoms of the patient so you can help him pinpoint the things that are making him ill and avoid them.
Do demonstrate your willingness to cooperate so the patient will do likewise.

4 *Don't* forget that the patient frequently has cerebral reactions which may prevent him from making necessary decisions.
Do remember that the patient often cannot remember to take relief measures at the time he needs them most.
Do remind the patient to take any prescribed treatment, such as oxygen, salts, neutralization therapy, etc.
Do remind the patient to drink water, take exercise, and take other measures that help alleviate reactions.
Do recognize that chemical, as well as food, reactions often set off

food addictions. When the patient is reacting, gently but firmly help him follow his diet. This may be a good time to encourage the patient to skip a meal, but only if this practice has been approved by his doctor.

A WORD OF CAUTION *Do remember* if the patient becomes annoyed and irritated with suggestions that might help him and he vehemently disclaims that he is reacting, it usually confirms the need for help. Proceed with a little gentle insistence and with a great deal of understanding.

Where to Take a Firm Stand

There are circumstances under which only a very firm stand by extremely sensitive persons will remind one and all of the seriousness of environmental illness. No compromise can be made under these conditions, and none should be expected. Be sure to notify tradespeople or family visitors that these are restrictions necessary for your health.

SMOKING While it would be best for everyone to give up smoking, if that is not possible, be firm and set these restrictions: no smoking in your presence; no smoking in your house; and no smoking in your car.

SMOKE ON CLOTHES If family members do smoke, or if they work with smokers, ask them to remove their clothes when they come home. The clothes should be placed in the basement, laundry room, or some place where they won't make you ill. The smoker or family member exposed to smoking should shower and wash his hair to remove the smoke that adheres to the body and hair.

PERFUMES ARE TOXIC Be firm about restricting the use of all perfumed products as well as products in aerosol cans.

The Importance of Support Groups

To be complete, your environmental education should include active membership in a support group. The two avenues of participation open to you are of equal importance: membership in the national and local organizations.

The national organization is The Human Ecology Action League (HEAL). Membership in this organization is important because it attracts national attention to your illness. It is the vehicle to educate the public, the government, and medical professionals who have not yet learned the techniques and value of clinical ecology. Your membership helps national HEAL present a united front against those who feel threatened by our movement and wish to destroy it.

A more tangible help offered by HEAL is their publication, "The Human Ecologist," which will be the source of your continuing environmental education. At the end of this book you will find a facsimile of the HEAL application. We suggest that you use the information to join the organization.

The second organization, but of equal importance to you, is the local support group. Some of these groups are local chapters of HEAL; others have only a loose affiliation with HEAL. Either way, national HEAL will help you find a local group. If there is none in your area, they will send you instructions on how to start a new chapter.

To help you understand the value of joining, we are including the following article that appeared in a HEAL newsletter. It was written by Natalie Golos, co-author of this book.

SUPPORT GROUPS: A TWO-WAY STREET

Some people are compulsive givers; some, compulsive takers. Neither approach is healthy and with neither can you receive realistic help from any support group, especially one for environmental illness. The givers burn themselves out; the takers learn bad habits of negativity and dependency.

In the foreword to *Coping With Your Allergies*, Dr. Randolph wrote, "One of the most troublesome tasks of practicing clinical ecology is the tremendous time required in the education of patients...." That is why so many books have been written on the subject and why so many support groups have been formed.

Education at its best is give and take: you learn by giving and you learn by taking. To strengthen our support group, I have been asked to share with you some painful memories of my educational process in environmental illness.

In 1966, when I returned from Dr. Randolph's hospital, I could not have survived without the Environmental Health Association (EHA), which was later replaced by HEAL. EHA had been formed three months earlier for the patients of Dr. Kailin, our clinical ecologist. It is no exaggeration to say that, with the help of Dr. Kailin and her staff, EHA members gave my life new direction and new purpose. I had to learn every new detail: what to eat and how to cook it; what to wear and where to buy it; how to build and furnish my house and which products to use for cleaning and maintaining it.

In the beginning my condition deteriorated as the polluted environment in each house forced me to move from place to place, seven times to be exact. Clinical ecology was in its infancy, without patient manuals and without the expertise and efficiency of today's methods. You, new patients, today are the beneficiaries of our trials and errors.

I was a taker, and people like Idris Newbill, the Ireys, and others were the givers. I told Dr. Kailin I was unable to go to EHA meetings because I was too sick to make the effort and my vision, too impaired for me to drive. In addition, I was afraid of the contamination of the meeting place. Dr. Kailin convinced me that the advantages far outweighed the disadvantages; social contact and the interchange with other patients were vital to a healthy positive mental attitude.

To enable me to come, the Ireys or the Ligons drove me to the meetings. So, I was a taker, but I was a giver too. To my surprise, it was from my giving that I received the most help.

From the onset of my illness, my greatest complaint was the trauma of going from the pleasure of a very active professional and social life to the misery of pain and discomfort in almost total isolation. Within three weeks of my return from the hospital, Dr. Kailin convinced me to assume an active role in EHA. I became membership chairman with the responsibility for counseling the patients. It was a natural for me because I was confined to my house, always available to receive calls. Except in emergencies, the patients called me with the questions. That helped Dr. Kailin by reducing the number of calls to her office; it helped the patients because, through me, they could find their answers without waiting for their next office visit.

Gradually I learned that most of the questions were environmental in nature and were repetitious. My calls to Dr. Kailin decreased, because I could answer many questions from previously learned information. Yes, I was a giver, but I was a taker too. From the patients I learned many of their own discoveries that helped me personally (new sources, new recipes, new helpful hints, etc.). From Dr. Kailin's answers for others, I sometimes stumbled onto a solution for one of my own complaints. This effort, with Dr. Kailin's help, finally launched me into the authorship of the first clinical ecology patient manual and, eventually, my other books.

Mine is not an isolated case. From contact with thousands of patients I have heard similar stories over and over again. The most susceptible patients received the greatest help by extending themselves for others. Such activity is therapeutic in its very diversion. Conversely, inactivity breeds self-indulgence, hopelessness, a sense of self pity, and a negative attitude that defeats any positive treatments. It is too detrimental to become totally self-absorbed. We have found a correlation between inactivity and increased sensitivity.

Even the healthy spouse, parent, or other family member of the patient has much to gain from active membership in the support group. This has usually proven to strengthen marriages and family ties at a time when illness can be a destructive force. By working and sharing with others in a similar situation, you can discover how others have learned to cope with the relative's illness. You can learn how and when to compromise and how to help create and nurture a positive attitude in a family where such support is sorely needed. In addition, you will be amazed how such activity on your part will be therapeutic for the patient, speeding the process of recovery and lightening your load.

In summary, a support group is a sharing group. Share your ideas, your information, and the responsibility for keeping your support group a viable thriving community. Join a committee! Take an active role! Don't wait! The next person you help may be yourself!

A Final Word

"To remain healthy in spite of physical discomfort and medical problems takes concentration and willpower. Yet, it is of paramount importance because so much of your future well-being depends on it." You may remember this quotation from the beginning of Chapter 30 of *Coping With Your Allergies*.

Nothing you will ever have to do will require more of the *total you* than overcoming your environmental illness. You have read about the need to squelch self-pity and you have been urged *to do something* in your own behalf. That's what this course is all about—to get you started or continue your efforts in the right direction to wellness.

In the same chapter on mental attitude, the authors went on with further advice that is worth repeating here.

Living with multiple allergies is not dull and it need not be depressing. Again, it all depends on your mental attitude and willingness to try something new. . . .

Fight illness with what might be called the "buddy system." If you are one who reacts to excitants by experiencing depression, it is important to have someone to help you. Because problems do not always conform to the office hours of professionals, you must sometimes turn to the nonprofessional. Friends and relatives seldom can be of any help because they cannot fully understand what they have not experienced—they tend to aggravate the condition by suggesting it is all in the mind.

Choose a buddy from the organization HEAL. When you call in tears and says, "Make me laugh," your buddy will immediately understand. "Make me laugh" is a password, because it eloquently expresses the basis of the person-to-person "buddy therapy." Of all the bromides applicable to patients, probably the most useful is, "laughter is the best medicine."

Your education has just begun. In essence, the main goal of this course has been to teach you how to educate yourself: to understand ecologic illness, to understand your own state of health, and to know how to plan your own lifestyle in order to reach an optimum state of good health.

Proceed at your own pace. Use as much of the program as you wish to or are able to. After you have completed the required and optional reading, turn to the Table of Contents in each of the books studied during the course. Check the books for other information that might be useful to you.

If you are at home, taking this course under the supervision of a doctor, turn to Part III, Class Six lesson plan for further guidance. If you still have questions, consult with the physician's staff member who is supervising your education.

PART II

How to Teach Environmental Medicine

Introduction to Counseling the Patient

In the Foreword to *Coping With Your Allergies*, Dr. Theron Randolph states:

One of the most troublesome tasks of practicing clinical ecology is the tremendous time required in the education of patients. The word *education* is used advisedly because more than instruction and question answering is involved. Patients must be educated in both the philosophy and distinctive features of this type of medicine as well as in the details of applying it.

With this need in mind, the authors have organized this book to give the ecology patient the necessary education and encouragement to help himself in assessment and analysis of his problems, and to provide practical guidance in coping with them. As the patient becomes more supportive of himself, the clinical ecologist, of course, is free to spend his time on medical rather than educational matters. Part I is primarily directed to the student/patient. Parts II and III are primarily for the counselor who is conducting this course at the direction of the clinical ecologist.

Some students/patients may not be able to participate in a traditional class setting and must conduct their own course at home. For this reason, the student has occasionally been directed to read in Parts II and III of this book. As we have done so before, we caution the student taking this course without benefit of a counselor to seek and follow closely the advice of your physician.

Successful Teaching

Adults invariably remember "outstanding" teachers. They were knowledgeable, organized, prepared, and dedicated. Good teaching is hard to define, but we do know it includes: motivation, goals, methods, knowledge, techniques of presentation, and skill in evaluating.

Motivation

The overriding motivation for the students is the physical benefit they will receive from their instruction and changed habits. Success or the anticipation of it will spur the student on in his pursuit of a healthier life. We believe we have built a good deal of motivation into Part I of this book, but it remains for the counselor to charge his discussion with encouragement many times during each lesson. There is a good deal to be gained by stating over and over that "success breeds success" and that "progress is worth the effort."

In the first of the counselor's lesson plans, we are setting an example of how to use motivation by motivating you, the counselor. From time to time in the procedural outlines, we will give you ideas to stimulate and maintain motivation, but be on the alert for the opportunities to build on the interests and contributions of the patients. Encourage spontaneity in group discussions, where the slightest spark may ignite others to persevere and succeed.

Make sure you review the patients' assignments in class. They should never feel that the reading was unnecessary or the testing unimportant. Review the lists they compile as well as the patients' answers to the questions. The patients should know they will have the opportunity to ask any questions if they don't understand something.

Every assignment should be reviewed. Review can take many forms and need not simply be a recitation of "correct" answers. For example, during Class One, it might be a good idea to show the pictures of the allergic faces in Doris Rapp's book and have group members look at each other to see if they can pick out some allergic faces. Another example: Start a class discussion by asking the patients if, after reading the first chapters of *If This Is Tuesday, It Must Be Chicken*, any of them have made changes such as finding wholesome substitutes for· sugar and salt. Or you may ask how many of them have been able to do away with the five worst offenders. When you review patients' work, do it from the point of view of what they have learned and how they are applying it. As the class sees how some of the people are applying what they are learning, they will be encouraged to try similar applications.

Motivation of the Teacher

In Part I, the objectives of the course are spelled out in the Introduction. Not surprisingly, because health is at stake, the objectives provide the motivation for the patient. The counselor, of course, is also motivated by the goal of good health for the patient. But there are specific and different motivations for the counselor. The counselor is a professional and like other professionals takes pride and satisfaction in doing his job well. The counselor recognizes the importance of his job and the high humanitarian contribution that he is making to society. This is especially clear to him because of the common denominator of that "society"—they are hurting and *need* him. Beyond his professionalism, the counselor sees a most unusual opportunity for a full expression of his humanness.

Practically speaking, for a job well done the counselor may see the opportunity for advancement. This becomes more a reality every day as there is an increased demand for competent teachers to instruct the support staffs of other doctors.

Importance of the Counselor's Role

The very business of weaning the patient away from the doctor and helping him establish his independence is the job of the counselor. He is not acting as a doctor; his role is *apart* from the doctor—between the doctor and the patient. The patients should see this early on in their education as the counselor guides and monitors them to better health and a freer life. The patient will see rather quickly how his medical costs are being reduced. The patient will benefit in yet another way—he will have the satisfaction of doing for himself.

Should these special values be pointed out to the patient who is less aware of the counselor's influence? Yes, by all means! Through the patient a larger world will learn of the contributions the counselor makes. A larger world will learn, as well, of the many advantages and blessings of the clinical ecology approach to the medical ministry. The patient can be the best advocate for environmental medicine as he speaks of the counselor with admiration and gratitude.

The counselor can serve as an adviser to the patient or patients who form support systems. He will assist them particularly in their efforts to create local chapters of HEAL. This is yet another way that the counselor helps the patient to develop confidence and independence. Of course, his role as instructor in the practices discussed in this book is the most prominent facet of his professional work. In this he is teacher and healer.

It has been said before that the patient who helps himself as prescribed in this course will free the doctor for more medically oriented pursuits. The counselor can well be the instrument by which this change is started. And the doctor and environmental medicine in general benefit. The more efficient use of the doctor's time is in itself a cost efficiency. The doctor will have more satisfied patients. He will have more enthusiastic patients. He will have more patients.

Goals

The objectives for each Class should serves as mileposts for the counselor. Instruction should be designed so that the student will have achieved the objective at some point in the class session. The goal of the counselor, then, is the achievement of the student/patient. By rephrasing the objectives into one or more questions, the counselor can determine the progress of the student. As in all group situations, the students can help each other learn through their questions and answers. A goal of the counselor, then, is to encourage this kind of cross-pollination by leading provocative discussions in class.

The learning formula most likely to be employed in this course is easily analyzed. *Knowledge* (from the readings) plus *experience* (of counselor and patient) is *presented* (in class assignments) and *evaluated* (through discussion and question-and-answer sessions) for *life goals* (improved health of patients and improved teaching skills of counselor). To achieve his personal goal of guiding the student/patient to improved health, the counselor must examine the elements of this formula in advance and have readied himself for all student sessions. A few tips may be helpful here.

KNOWLEDGE Counselor will certainly read the basic books thoroughly and will know the relationship of *each assignment to the entire course.* Counselor will have read other works in the bibliography and have assimilated their information with his professional training.

EXPERIENCE Counselor should have appropriate notes of his personal experiences, of case studies, from other readings to supplement the information in this book, and the assigned readings. Counselor should strongly encourage student/patients to share their experiences in class sessions. Counselor can then add to his stockpile of useful, relevant information for future courses.

PRESENTATION Counselor should follow sequence of classes, but will know when certain objectives require additional attention. The "Preview" for each session is important, as students want to know the parameters of each Class. The "Preview" gives the counselor the best chance to spot the more difficult aspects of a particular class assignment, where explanation is necessary. In the presentation (discussion and questions and answers) counselor should always remember that *the patient is interested in applying the information to his problem.* Every effort should be made to see that this happens. On occasions, referrals will have to be made to the physician who is overseeing the course—but attempts should be made to resolve all problems cooperatively. The patient should not be left to solve problems on his own. The counselor should summarize the major points of each Class and each Class should be briefly reviewed in subsequent discussions. Briefer and briefer reviews in subsequent sessions will provide a repetition that spirals upward throughout the course.

EVALUATION   Counselor is continually evaluating (measuring) the success of the course. Correct answers to questions and richer, more meaningful discussions are indications that real progress is being made. Heightened interest in the course, more confidence on the part of students, and actual behavioral changes are evidence of success. The counselor should look for these signs and encourage students when they exhibit them.

LIFE GOALS   Counselor knows from the foregoing section on motivation that gratification will be postponed. A lifetime of better living cannot be telescoped or otherwise shown to student or counselor. Satisfaction comes to both of them with a few steps in the directions of improvement, *day by day*.

Tips for the New Teacher

Every teacher adds to his arsenal of techniques with each classroom session. The education of the teacher literally goes on and on. These few suggestions, then, are to start you on the way to making your personal list of techniques:

1 Until you have gained experience through conducting several classes, review all materials, cross-references, and sources. You will gain confidence knowing what is available. If you don't know the answers to certain questions, be sure to let the class know you will make every effort to find the information if it is available.

2 A good teacher checks in advance to see that the classroom is in good condition (i.e., clean, well lit, well ventilated, well heated or cooled, etc.).

3 For each class, you must check that the necessary books, pencils, papers, blackboard, chalk, and any other materials are available.

4 Begin each class with new material, when the students are fresh enough to absorb it.

5 Whenever the class lags, take a break. Have the students stretch, walk around, do some breathing exercises, and get something to drink.

6 Allow yourself enough time to review the previous assignment.

7 Be sure to give complete instructions for the next assignment.

8 Whenever there is extra time, practice developing a rotary diversified diet or have a question-and-answer period.

Do's and Don'ts for the Group Counselor

1 DON'T give medical advice except when suggested by the
supervising doctor.
NEVER recommend a medication or treatment of any kind.
NEVER suggest even those medical practices that are used successfully
by most patients.
    Example 1: The alkali salts are not safe for everyone, especially
patients with kidney or heart problems.
    Example 2: Oxygen is sometimes contraindicated.
DO refer all medical questions to the doctor.

2 DON'T let one patient monopolize the session with personal
problems.
DO suggest a private consultation with you or the doctor.
DO keep the discussion general and of interest to all.

3 DON'T be rigid with your lesson plans.
DO try to adhere to your plans, but be flexible. If you intend to
cover one area but the patients need help in another,
accommodate their requests. You can easily return to your topic
later on in the next session.

4 DON'T give the impression that any one of the tests or treatments
is the only acceptable method.
DO remember that patients may be on different diets. Some may
be on the rotary diversified mono-food diet; others may just be
rotating foods. Some may be on the Rowe diet or similar
elimination diet.
DO remember that some patients may be on avoidance only;
some on injections; some on drops; and some on a combination.
DO remember that the same is true for chemicals.
DO remember that some patients are managing complex allergies;
others have mild chemical sensitivities and are interested
primarily in prevention.
(CAUTION: Remind patients that, whenever possible, excitants must
be avoided. For example: injections for dust sensitivity are not
a license to live in a dust-filled room.)

5 DON'T conduct the session as a lecture.
DO let the session be a group activity. Encourage the patients to
discuss products they can tolerate, but remind the group that
no product is safe for everyone. Every product must be tested by
the extremely sensitive patient.

6 DON'T recommend anything as *safe*, not even something in one of
your source books.
DO recommend that sensitive patients test everything before
using it for the first time.
DO remind patients that any product intended for a large surface
area should be tested first on something that can be removed
from the house. Test it a few times in increasingly larger areas.

Even when you think it is safe, first apply it in a small room. Tell the group that something seemingly safe on a small surface sometimes proves unsafe in larger areas.

7 DON'T let negative attitudes prevail. Never let one negative patient dominate the scene.

DO encourage personal testimonies, enabling patients to exchange ideas and viewpoints. This will help them learn how to improve their general well-being.

DO let patients briefly voice negative viewpoints. It is important to let them voice their discouragement.

DO turn the negative to a positive by telling about patients who were worse and who were also discouraged, but who are so much better now.

DO remind the most discouraged that even if they can't do everything, doing something is better than doing nothing.

    Example 1: If a patient can't change the entire house, he should concentrate on one or two rooms.

    Example 2: If a patient can't change his environment, he should be more careful with his diet, his clothes, and his activities.

    Example 3: If a patient can't change everything at once, he should select priorities and make gradual changes.

DO remind the patient that indulging in self-pity will not, for example, get rid of the carpet in his rented home but can aggravate his reaction to it.

DO remind the patients of the importance of stress management.

8 DON'T put limits on precautions to be taken.

DO suggest that the greater the number of precautions taken, the sooner the patient will begin to build tolerance and improve his adaptability, regardless of how mild or how severe his sensitivity.

DO encourage caution with chemicals even for those who test negative to chemical sensitivities, reminding them that it is wiser to prevent complex sensitivities than to risk having to deal with them at a later time.

9 DON'T put any pressure on the patients.

DO remember that they already have more stress than they can handle.

DO remember that many patients suffer from cerebral edema and recurring learning disabilities.

DO keep reminding them that they have the tools to refresh their memories.

DO remind them to keep their class questionnaires for future reference.

DO keep assuring them they don't have to remember everything, just where to find their answers.

DO, above all, remember that mental confusion and behavioral manifestations are often caused by their illness, so BE PATIENT!!

PART III

Lesson Plans

PRECLASS INSTRUCTIONS

After the physician has made the decision to educate the patient, the counselor should meet with the patient.

1 Be sure that the patient understands his initial instructions.

2 Be sure that the patient understands the importance of education.

3 Explain the structure of the course for patients as well as its objectives:

- To save money.
- To save time.
- To meet others for support.
- To help the people on a waiting list to begin helping themselves.
- To learn to assume greater responsibility for one's own health.

4 Explain the cost of the class, the payment plan, and how to substitute for missed sessions, and the availability of additional private sessions.

5 Sign the patient up for the course or instruct the patient that he will be notified when there is an opening.

6 See that the patient has copies of the textbook and basic reading list. If they don't already have the hardcover, recommend the paperback which is usually a revised updated version.

7 Discuss the importance of doing assignments. Turn to "Assignment for Class One." Instruct the patient to read the material carefully everything that is in Class One as well as the assigned reading in the other books.

8 Instruct the patient to bring all materials, including books and assignments, to all classes.

9 Indicate that the course consists of six sessions, each one lasting between one and two hours.

10 Be sure that the class members understand that, in six lessons, it would be impossible to cover all the material recommended in the book. These are only suggestions to guide the class to continuing their education on their own. After their testing and course work are finished, patients will become their own counselors. This is how to reduce the risk involved in *self-help*.

11 Mention that the group is sometimes given optional reading material that has already been covered in a different way. For example, the rotary diversified diet is covered in *If This Is Tuesday, It Must Be Chicken*, but for optional reading there is coverage in *Coping With Your Allergies*, and in *An Alternative Approach to Allergies*. If he has no chance to read these optional assignments while the course is in progress, he should do so when it is over. Education in the field of environmental medicine is a continuing process for the patient.

Lesson Plan for Class One

I.   Have class members introduce themselves. Discuss any personal experiences they have had where education would have helped. Tell them that they will be limited to two minutes. Time each person to prevent him from rambling on.

  A.   The participants have been instructed to read Class One and its assignments before the first session. With this in mind, spend a few minutes discussing why this was recommended and why this class is so important to them. Discuss why it is important for the class members to have enough knowledge to educate other people with whom they have contact. For example, when asking a tradesperson to do something out of the ordinary, patients must have enough knowledge to be able to explain their requests properly. Knowledge will result in more cooperation if the tradesperson does not think the patient is eccentric.

  B.   Discuss a good way to organize *If This Is Tuesday, It Must Be Chicken*. This can be done by purchasing different color tabs and securing them to the title page of Chapters 7, 8, 9, and 10. This way the patient can quickly turn to the rotation desired.

  C.   Tell the patients that priority should be given to reading the assigned material because it was prepared specifically for this course.

  D.   Refer to "Objectives of the Course" and "Course Design" in Part I of the textbook. It is important to tell class members what they are studying and why. This is a good place to assure the class that the object of this course is to teach participants how to help themselves, that they are not expected to remember everything.

II.   Ask if there are any questions about Assignment One. A sample question could be: "From your assignment, what did you learn about allergies that surprised you?" Refer to Dr. Rapp's book, pages 67 and 68 for atypical allergy symptoms.

A. Lead the patients in a discussion of pages 126–127 of Dr. Rapp's book. Reinforce the point that these foods do not always cause allergies and that foods listed as seldom causing allergies will nonetheless be allergenic to some people.

B. It is important to emphasize that medical problems *identified* as being caused by foods are not always caused by foods. It is important to emphasize and reemphasize that the foods listed as causing hives are not the only things that cause hives. However, it is wise for the person who constantly has hives, to go without the suspected causes for a period of ten days to see if the hives clear up. If he is not willing to omit the whole list of possible causes at once, he can omit them one at a time. If the hives clear up, then he can be fairly sure he has found the culprit. If they do not, he can methodically go through the whole list. Or, he can eliminate all the things that are on the list, see if the hives clear up, and if they do clear up, he can then reintroduce them one at a time. Discuss these two procedures for testing.

C. *Discrepancy:* On Page 126, under "Related Foods," Dr. Rapp says that wheat and buckwheat are in no way related to each other. However, buckwheat is a known sensitizer and thus should be used only once weekly by the wheat sensitive patient.

III. Lead a brief discussion of the precautions class members have initiated since reading Class One.

IV. Remind the class members to keep all of their materials together (including their assignments) and to bring them all to class for each session.

V. Discuss the assignment for Class Two to insure that class members know which chapters to read. Don't be afraid to discuss that there are differing opinions and approaches.

I. Before Teaching the Rotary Diversified Diet (RDD)

A. You must carefully study all the cross references on foods. Because a RDD must be individual, it is advisable to schedule a private session for each food-sensitive patient. Nevertheless, it is important to teach the mechanics of planning a diet. From time to time, people have to change their diet for variety or out of necessity as they lose or gain new foods. Even if a class member is not currently rotating foods, emphasize the importance of understanding the concept.

B. You must be careful to chose the rotary diversified diet format that fits into your doctor's practice. If he does not want patients to repeat any food family for four days, that is what you must teach. Therefore, because doctors may differ in their approach, this is going to vary from office to office. However, we will present all the ideas so that the physician can decide whether he wants to give the patients a choice or whether he is going to require his patients to do it one specific way. Whatever he decides, it is always good to know that there are variations. In the same way that a doctor can choose from among different medications (i.e., different anthistamines or different antibiotics), he can choose from different variations of the rotary diversified diet.

C. You must consider variables in addition to those given to the patient.

1. Even those patients who are candidates for very stringent methods may not be quite ready for drastic changes in their eating habits. Always approach the topic, especially in the beginning, from the point of view of choice, the point of view of prevention. Don't scare them off. You can mention that those people who already realize they have complex chemical susceptibility would be wise to use the Rinkle/Randolph method which follows. Later, after Class Three, when the group has completed the Chemical Questionnaire, more class members will be convinced to follow this stricter approach. The doctor will make the final decision as to which course of action is most suitable for each patient.

2. If the RDD is being used as a diagnostic tool, you must consider whether it is the sole form of testing or if it is being supplemented with other tests, such as an elimination diet, provocative testing, or RAST testing, etc.

3. It has to be the doctor's decision when to take the ecologically-oriented history and whether he wants the patient to keep a diary that includes a record of all foods eaten one or two weeks prior to testing. If the RDD is the sole form of testing, in order for it to be at all valid, it must be composed of one food per meal, repeated for a minimum of three cycles, and not interchangeable with other foods of the same family. To limit the problem of delayed reactions, only one suspected food should be used per day.

4. The formula in *If This Is Tuesday, It Must Be Chicken* was devised so that with very little knowledge a patient will be able to make his own diet changes. Therefore, even technicians with years of practice with the RDD might be wise to learn how to use the formula so they can teach it to the patient.

When the diet is used for treatment, most patients eventually use multiple food meals. There are varying degrees of rotation discussed in *If This Is Tuesday, It Must Be Chicken:*

a. Permitting the dieter to eat any food (or member of that food family) all day long provided none is repeated for a four-day cycle, e.g., cherries, almonds, and peaches all day long.

b. Restricting the intake of any food to one meal in the four-day cycle but permitting eating the related foods during the same day, e.g., almonds for breakfast, cherries for lunch, peaches for dinner.

c. Limiting the patient to only one meal from an entire food family during the whole four-day cycle, e.g., almonds, cherries, and/or peaches all at one meal and not repeated again during the four-day cycle (Rinkle/Randolph rotary diversified diet).

Before we discuss the fourth variation, we want to mention that Dr. Randolph requested that we make the following statement: The Rinkle/Randolph rotation does not encompass #1 and #2 and he does not recommend them. We offer them as alternatives, here, and in *If This Is Tuesday, It Must Be Chicken* because they were requested by other doctors. Some doctors use these variations in order to provide a greater variety for the patients as they begin the process and are easing into rotation. Additionally, those doctors wanted #1 and #2 for people interested in prevention of food allergies and for healthy members of families prone to allergy. The book clearly states which menus adhere strictly to the Rinkle/Randolph rotation, and which do not.

The fourth variation which involves dividing food families is not discussed in *If This Is Tuesday, It Must Be Chicken* because it was found that patients created problems for themselves, losing many foods, as a result of combining the different variations. After the patient understands all the pitfalls of the fourth variation, suggest that he use it only under close supervision by you or the doctor.

d. In the fourth variation the food families can be divided into related foods to be eaten on alternate days, e.g., apples on Monday and pears on Wednesday, or wheat on Monday and rice on Wednesday. It must be the doctor's decision if and how the foods are to be divided because there are some concommitant foods, i.e., during the season when an inhalant is a problem, a food may also be a problem. There are also some synergistic foods, i.e., foods that cause problems when ingested together even if they do not cause problems when eaten alone.

If the doctor decides to use this variation, it can be done with the numbering system in *If This Is Tuesday, It Must be Chicken*, by labeling some foods in one family x and some y. Do not use *a, b* or *c*, because they have already been used to divide the #40 Rose family (see page 111) into pomes, stone fruits, berries and herbs. Thus, the 40b group could be further subdivided:

40b stone fruits:

| x almonds | y peach (nectarine) |
| x apricots | y plum (prune) |

Cherries could be labeled x or y according to the availability of the fruit.

Another example of the subdivision could be family #45, citrus. For example, grapefruit could be an x and orange a y. In examples such as these, you must be careful to place oranges, tangerines and tangelos all in the same subdivision because the latter are said to be hybrids of the two former fruits.

An example of the need for caution is the division of grains. You cannot have wheat on Monday and rye on Wednesday. Some physicians believe that all grains with gluten must be eaten on the same day, leaving the other grains for the alternate day. In fact, some doctors believe that all grains should be eaten on one day.

A further example for caution in subdividing the foods is that it limits the use of recipes and menus in *If This Is Tuesday, It Must Be Chicken*.

If your doctor decides to use the fourth variation, here are three suggestions that will simplify the process for the patient:

i. Divide only those families where it is a hardship not to do so, e.g., not enough green vegetables, not enough fruit in the off season, not enough safe foods (non-allergy foods) in the diet.

ii. Be sure that the patient draws up a new food chart for each day, incorporating the subdivisions in the charts and menus (see pages 118–121).

   iii. Be sure the patient makes corrections in the list of food families, pages 109–117.

   Caution: Be sure the patient is advised to check each recipe to see that he is not inadvertently repeating a vegetable.

   Example: Let us say that he is putting green peppers on Day 1 and tomatoes on Day 3. Explain that he cannot make the basic stuffed pepper with the tomato juice in it (see page 51 *If This Is Tuesday, It Must Be Chicken*) unless he uses the formula to omit the tomatoes for one cycle.

D. Once the doctor has decided which approach to use for the RDD treatment, you can teach patients how to plan their own diets. Since repetition is a good teaching tool, always have the patient use the same approach.

   1. Alphabetize the safe foods or the allergens, whichever is fewer in number.

   2. Plan the diet following the charts for Days 1 through 4 (see pages 118–121).

      a. In the event that there are not enough foods, the patient can add his minus-ones (–1) and plus ones (+1).

      b. If necessary, the patient can add exotic, untested foods.

   3. Using the formula, with the patient's cooperation, switch food families for combinations acceptable to the patient.

   4. When necessary, divide the food family for every other day.

      a. Insure avoiding the combination of techniques.

      b. Use the procedure preferred by the physician.

E. You must discuss related and unrelated foods. Mention that it is possible to have a sensitivity to one food and have no problem with others of the same family, i.e., allergic to apples but not pears. In such a case, the patient would be wise to avoid pears as well as apples for a few months. However, if he has so few compatible foods that he needs pears in his diet, he should space the pears at least a week or two apart. This arrangement applies to other food families, especially the grain and legume families.

II. Teaching the RDD in Class.

A. Explain the reasons the patients must know how to plan a diet. Explain that it takes a few practice tries and then it comes as second nature.

B. Be sure that everyone understands the alphabetical and numerical lists.

C. Have the class turn to Appendix B, pages 118–121. On page 118, discuss "Food Families Used," indicated by number. Discuss the numbers of the animal protein, vegetables, etc.

D. Using one patient's list of food allergens, locate the days from which the food must be eliminated.

E. Follow through by planning the patient's diet, using the formula if necessary.

F. Emphasize the fact that in the beginning, whenever patients go on rotation, they receive help planning the diet. However, it is necessary to understand the process so they can make future changes with ease.

G. Mention that *Coping With Your Allergies*, P pages 83–107 and 137–166 or H pages 75–98 and 127–151, presents a more comprehensive discussion about food. Emphasize the fact that these procedures have been written for the patients extremely food sensitive and chemically susceptible. It is the approach necessarily strict for this those who have recently been in a hospital ecology unit or are ill enough to be candidates for hospitalization. It is important for everyone to know all aspects of this dietary program. They will also want to read about food allergy in *An Alternative Approach to Allergies.*

III. Explain the reason for the section on 'Yeast' in Class Two (taken from Chapter 11 of *Coping With Your Allergies*). It is important to know about the foods containing yeast, molds, and malt that sometimes cause problems for people with allergies. Until such time as they learn whether or not this is their problem, it is wise to cut down on yeast and mold foods. Chemically-susceptible and food-allergic people do not need the stress of additional yeast and mold foods. Here, emphasize "Don't try to be a 100 percenter." Tell them that they can approach it by taking away some of the foods to see if it improves their health. If they find relief by giving up all cheeses, for example, then they should give up additional mold foods. If they find that by giving up pasteurized fruit juices they feel better, then they should avoid other yeast foods. In other words, this is just a slight introduction. Don't overwhelm them with an in-depth discussion of candidiasis or the use of nystatin.

At this point we wish only to introduce it in passing. Since there is now so much talk about candidiasis and since there are so many who are involved with nystatin, some questions may be raised by a class member. If so, it is important to say that this is an individual problem best discussed in a private session with the doctor. Say that the entire subject will be covered in a future session.

IV Closing Procedure

A. Ask if there are any questions, still unanswered, from the assignment for Class Two.

B. Introduce the section, "Saving Money." Ask members for their suggestions for additional ways to save money using environmentally safe methods. Tell them that the discussion on cleaning refers only to saving money. Class three will have a very thorough discussion of cleaning.

C. Collect the lists of alphabetical food allergies so you can check to see if class members clearly understand the numbering systems.

D. Have the students turn briefly to the assignment for class three.

E. See that each class member has a copy of *An Alternative Approach to Allergies*. Have them turn to the Randolph questionnaire form, pointing out how it is used and why it is important to complete it. Suggest that if they wish to be objective, they first answer all questions without reading the explanations. Have them turn to P page 224 or H page

189 and guide them through the chapter pointing out the the explanatory sections that they should ignore for the time being.

After they have finished answering the questions, they should read the section in the textbook entitled "Interpreting the Questionnaire." At that point, they can read Chapter 19 in *An Alternative Approach to Allergies.* Then they can go back over their answers. If they suspect that they are chemically susceptible, suggest an appointment for a private session with you or, if possible, a consultation with the physician.

Lesson Plan for Class Three

I. Conduct a practice session working with the diet. This time, choose a patient other than one who participated in the last class. Have all the patients help design the diet.

II. Because Class Three is so important make certain that you have enough time to discuss it in class. Of course, continue the discussion in future classes as it is necessary.

A. Lead the class in a discussion on the questionnaire. Ask how many people now believe they have some chemical sensitivities. Then ask how many people think they have mild chemical sensitivities. Then ask how many think they have severe chemical sensitivities.

B. Have them turn to P page 227 or H page 191 in *An Alternative Approach to Allergies*. Point out the division of groups: the main category of the first group is "Coal, Oil, Gas, & Combustion Products." Have someone read aloud the first ten by-products. Explain the relationship between petroleum and the odor of fresh newspaper. If anyone has noted that he has become ill from several of the substances listed in the twenty-three questions in that group, he should seriously consider taking a test to see how he is affected by the gas stove. From the bottom of P page 228 or H page 192 he can learn to associate dry garbage incinerators with cold cream and hand lotions. If the patient becomes sick from the tarring of roofs and asphalt pavements, it may never have occurred to him that inks and carbons and the dyes in his shoes, cosmetics, and clothing could be bothering him. In other words, he may know he reacts to the worst form, but he probably does not suspect that he is also reacting to the minor forms because the symptoms are being masked. Additionally, even if his symptoms are evident, he frequently does not suspect the less noxious products like nonperfumed creams and lotions.

C. Spend enough time on the questionnaire to encourage the patients to study and know how to check out their own forms.

III. Have the class turn to the section of the textbook entitled "Cleaning." Introduce the subject of cleaning products and methods of cleaning.

A. Suggest that until their testing is completed, instead of using their current cleaning detergents, they use the following:

1. Baking soda

2. Neo-Life Organic Green, Rugged Red, and Dishwashing Detergent, as the manufacturer suggests.

3. Bon Ami Cake Soap and Bon Ami Cleaning Powder for heavy duty cleaning instead of cleansers like Ajax or Comet. Be sure to suggest the original *square* box of Bon Ami. The round box has toxic additives.

4. Pure apple cider vinegar.

B. Explain that these products are no more expensive to use and in many cases are less expensive. They are just as efficient and less toxic than most products on the market.

C. Be prepared to tell them where they can purchase these products locally or where to send away for them.

D. Ask if there are unanswered questions from the previous assignment. Have the class take turns reading from the lists they prepared while reading Chapter 4 of *Coping With Your Allergies.* Lead a discussion of changes and substitutions already made. Then ask how that chapter will affect future replacements.

E. Emphasize the fact that you don't expect them to be 100 percenters. Emphasize prevention. Downplay complex chemical sensitivity for the time being.

F. State that Chapter 24 in *Coping With Your Allergies* should be self-explanatory, as is the section entitled "Cleaning" in the textbook. Ask if there are any questions. Ask how many have tried any of the suggestions.

G. Encourage the class to practice stress reduction. Discuss meditation, biofeedback, or any other way to learn relaxation and proper breathing techniques.

H. Have the class turn to Assignment for Class Four. Briefly point out what they will be learning. Turn to the paper, "The Hypothesis of Immune System Dysregulation in Food and Chemical Sensitivities," by Dr. Alan S. Levin. Tell the class that the paper is one doctor's hypothesis, but it gives a clear understanding of the philosophy of environmental medicine. It is very important as you give the assignment to emphasize once again that they should not try to be a 100 percenter. Emphasize that their choices may very well be determined as a result of the Randolph questionnaire that they have answered for Class Three.

Lesson Plan for Class Four

I. Ask if there are any questions about the paper by Dr. Levin. Remind them that this is a hypothesis, which means that it is not to be accepted as gospel, but that clinical ecologists agree for the most part that this is a good explanation of food and chemical sensitivity.

    A. This paper describes chemical sensitivity, explains the immune system, furnishes information that patients can use to educate others but, most important, gives further motivation to the class. Take the time to have members read specific paragraphs from the early part of the paper through the immune stimulation techniques.

    B. Bring it to their attention that the course emphasizes a positive mental attitude and teaches how to manage stress by minimizing exposure and using the proper food in the context of healthful nutritional principles.

    C. The rest of Dr. Levin's recommendations must be supervised by a physician, i.e., harmful disease agents, immune stimulation techniques, and nutritional supplements.

II. Lead a discussion on home testing. See this section in Class Four.

    A. Patients will want to test things for different reasons:

        1. To test a food or chemical they suspect.

        2. To check products purchased on approval.

        3. To experiment with new untried or exotic foods in order to vary their diet.

        4. To re-evaluate foods and chemicals to see what progress has been made months after they were first tested by the physician.

    B. The simple home tests will not always be conclusive because the patient could have been exposed to a toxic chemical at the time of testing. Delayed reactions can also make tests invalid. Nevertheless, the tests may suffice until they can be verified by the doctor.

C. Emphasize how helpful it would be to the doctor if the patient has kept a diary during the home testing period. The diary should include a record of the time of the test, time of reactions, time of other foods eaten, and exposure to any toxic fumes. Of course, it should include the pulse and temperature readings as described in Class Four.

D. Discuss withdrawal, masking, and readaptation. Make sure the class understands why they must test a food within twelve days after avoidance. If readaptation has occurred, the remasking could make the test invalid.

III. Lead a discussion on the assigned material from *An Alternative Approach to Allergies.*

A. Turn to the addiction pyramid on P page 22 or H page 18 of *An Alternative Approach to Allergies.* Point out that addiction increases from slowly to more rapidly absorbed ingestants. (See the printing on the side of the diagram). For example, it moves from oils and fats, through proteins, through starches, and then through sugars. Thus, sugars are more quickly absorbed than starches, and the starches are more quickly absorbed than proteins. It is more likely that people will become addicted to sugars than they will to oils and fats. Moving up, teas, alcoholic beverages and cigarettes are the next level of addiction. Even farther up are drugs, finally moving into heroin at the top of the addiction pyramid.

B. Because it was a historical discovery and because it so aptly explains the masking process, refer to Dr. Rinkel's discovery on P page 23 or H page 19.

C. Turn to P page 38 or H page 30 in *An Alternative Approach to Allergies.* In detail, discuss the ups and downs of addiction as they apply to members of the class. Direct their attention to the top, where it says "start at zero, etc." Mention that homeostasis is the level of mood balance and good health. Show how plus one people can start the pattern up until it becomes a little more exaggerated, "hopped up." People who tend to become hyperactive start out by being very active, alert, and very enthusiastic.

Go through all the levels, having the class go through it very carefully to see where they belong. They will find that they are at different levels at different times. Indicate that this is the way for them to start studying their patterns. The person who is usually responsive, enthusiastic, lively and active most of the time but who from time to time is talkative, argumentative, sensitive, "hopped up," tense, and jittery is an example.

Show how the same people will go from a period of two plus to a period of two minus. Direct their attention to the very bottom of that page, underneath the line "cardiovascular manifestations, etc." to illustrate the relationship of allergy to the cardiovascular problem. Indicate that as a reason for taking the pulse rate to see if there is a change.

D. Mention that Chapters 8 through 13 in *An Alternative Approach to Allergies* delve more deeply into the withdrawal and stimulatory levels described on P page 38 or H page 30. However, spend a little time directing their attention to Chapter 11, P pages 139–145 or H pages 117–122 so they can check to see what type of reactions they have.

They should know the six major kinds of localized reactions and five main kinds of systemic withdrawal manifestations. This too is a further explanation of the charts. This knowledge is important for them to use as it applies to them. They will have a fairly good picture of how much they should do if they wish to return to better health. It is good motivation for them to follow certain restrictions that ordinarily they might not be willing to do.

IV. Closing Procedures

A. Ask the class if there are any unanswered questions from today's assignment.

B. Spend some time discussing the next assignment.

1. Chapters 17–23 and Chapters 26–30 in *Coping With Your Allergies* are assigned readings for Class Five. But reference to them is important at this time to point up the caution. The people who would be taking the kind

of test described in Chapter 17 would be those who are
obviously very chemically sensitive and therefore could
run into a great deal of difficulty. Thus, *this must be done
under the supervision of a doctor.* However, state that
all the patients should read the material so that they can
see which substances they will want to test individually
once they have read about simple testing methods.
Suggest that, before trying any tests, they carefully
review "Doing Your Own Testing." They can then do the
easy tests for individual products or procedures.
Encourage them to try two tests before the next class,
perhaps their drinking water and one food.

2. As the students read the assigned chapters for Class
Five in *Coping With Your Allergies,* they should be
thinking in terms of procedures they can use that will
cost little or no money. In addition, they should make a
list of things they will eventually want to replace.
Emphasize how these chapters can help them avoid
mistakes with future purchases and procedures, as well
as immediate changes. If they have their own copy of
the book, they can mark up the places, e.g., blue pencil
for immediate changes and red pencil for future changes.

I. This is a good time to discuss sources. Mention the fact that no sooner do we find a good source than one of two things may happen:

A. The source dries up. A good example of that is the International Hot Water Unit, recommended in the hard cover *Coping With Your Allergies* and in other ecology books. The company that made it is no longer in existence.

If a patient writes away for information and finds out that it is outdated, he should make a notation of that in his book so that he will know not to contact that company any more.

B. The manufacturer changes the product so that we can no longer use it. They should *not* take it for granted that any product that we mention is safe. They must test it on themselves, because not every product is safe for everyone. Nothing is recommended; rather, products that are listed in *Coping With Your Allergies* are products that have been used safely by at least ten or more extremely chemically-sensitive and food-sensitive patients.

Tell the class members that later in the course you will discuss the Bibliography that lists other sources. It is important at this time to recommend HEAL's publication, *The Human Ecologist*, as a good way to keep up with sources.

II. From the chapters assigned in *Coping With Your Allergies*, lead a discussion of those suggestions that the patients find practical for themselves. Here are some ideas that might make the discussion helpful.

A. It may not be possible to follow all the suggestions in Chapter 18, "How to Begin a Toxic-Free Life." However, any improvement is better than nothing. If they can't remove all the papers and books from the bedroom, they should at least attempt to put them in an enclosed bookcase or a galvanized garbage pail with a tight lid. For appearance sake, they can cover the pail with a pretty cotton cloth.

Carpeting in bedrooms can be a problem. Besides gathering dust, it becomes moldy. Even if patients are not sensitive to dust or molds, carpets are not advisable for allergy patients because of synthetic fibers or moth proofing. Whenever possible, it is better to sleep in a bedroom with bare floors. If you must have some floor covering, at least use a rug that can be removed, washed, and dried.

It should be emphasized that, regardless of the degree of sensitivity, in this modern world where chemicals are rampant, it is advisable that everyone have several hours a day in as pure an environment as possible. Since people spend six to eight hours sleeping, what better place to be pure than the bedroom.

B. Have the class turn to P page 186 or H page 170 and look over the suggestions. Tell them that no one can be expected to give up all the items listed. Once people are informed, they can begin to remove as many toxic products as possible from their environment. To illustrate, some people automatically use a felt-tip pen when they are writing nothing of importance. Because they are less toxic, metal ball point pens are better for important papers and for checks. Pencils can be used for other writing.

Toxic products like felt-tip pens can be harmful even to those who consider themselves healthy. A case in point describes how so called "experts" are frequently uninformed. At a task force mandated by Congress and conducted by several governmental health agencies, approximately one hundred people were invited to discuss the environmental impact on health. The co-author was there representing HEAL.

These were normally healthy people, doctors, nurses, and scientists called together to advise the government. In one of the rooms, people were beginning to show signs of discomfort. Not one of them even suspected the cause until the co-author explained it to the group.

The moderator had been using a toluene-based felt-tip pen to write suggestions on large sheets of paper which were then tacked up on the walls all around the room. Until it was called to their attention, many did not relate the overpowering fumes to the ill effects they were beginning to experience.

The next day the room was ventilated, the moderator switched to a water-based felt-tip pen, and people felt better. The moderator, an M.D., made a point of telling the author that he felt much better on the second day. He told her, "Yesterday I was 'hyped up' and didn't know why." Other members of the group also told her of their surprise at their reactions to the fumes from the toluene felt-tip pen.

There are two lessons to be learned from this experience. First, even so-called healthy, normal people react to toxic substances and so-called experts in the field (the people attending this conference were consultants on the environment's impact on health) do not associate their reactions with toxic substances.

You can use this experience to motivate the class to follow some of the suggestions in the assigned chapters. As an example, show that by carefully checking Chapter 19, they will learn some ways to avoid toxins.

C.   Ask how many people smell toilet tissue before they purchase it. Toilet tissue and facial tissue have varying degrees of formaldehyde (and/or perfume) in them. Why not use one that has no smell at all? You can point out that:

1.   The facial tissues and toilet tissues that have less odor usually are less toxic; and

2.   When a felt-tip pen is required, at least be sure to use a water-based one available in supermarkets and toy stores. Otherwise, use a metal ballpoint pen or a pencil.

D.   While Chapter 20, "Making Life Easier," is for the

extremely ill patient, nevertheless it is a good way to remind people that they can shop by telephone and that there are certain things they can do to make it easier to shop.

E.   Many patients have negative attitudes because they feel that it is too costly to make changes that will clean up their environment. To counteract that feeling, the motto, "Don't try to be a 100 percenter" was developed. Encourage them to search the literature for cost-free and inexpensive measures to help reduce their exposure to toxins.

Dr. Randolph disapproves of the negative connotation of the motto "Don't try to be a 100 percenter." In theory, we totally agree with him. We know that the rate of improvement of the patient correlates directly with the speed and the degree of environmental improvement.

Unfortunately, there are too many people who are discouraged from doing anything because they fear they can't do it all. The motto was intended to say to the patient, "Do the best you can." Meanwhile, those providing counseling should encourage more and more effort as time progresses. As the patient is educated, as he shows improvement from early changes, and as he learns to associate his symptoms with the environmental cause, it is our expectation that he will develop a more positive approach.

F.   Use Chapter 21, P page 200 or H page 182, as an illustration of the following: Wash your hair and clothes and take a shower after you have been exposed to a lot of chemicals so that you do not continue to breathe in all of the contaminants that you have been exposed to all day long. It is important to discuss spring-water enemas, as well. If patients are drinking spring water, they should not use tap water for an enema.

G.   Patients are always missing helpful hints because they assume that parts of the literature do not apply to them. Urge them to read everything because they will find things that apply to everyone.

   1.   They may ignore Chapter 23 because they are not

building a house. Even in an apartment, though, changes have to be made. For example, if the patient must put calking in his bathroom, he should use the old-fashioned caulking rather than the new silicon type. Class members should read this chapter even if, on the face of it, it does not seem to apply to them.

2.   A correction is needed for Chapter 23 in the hardcover. We have not found better paint than the DuPont Lucite Semi-Gloss Paint. Unfortunately, they are no longer making it without Teflon, but by adding baking soda to it, it is better than nothing, and better than most other paints. Make sure that the baking soda is mixed in thoroughly with the paint so that there are no lumps of baking soda because lumps will cause it to streak on the wall. Sift the baking soda, as you would flour for a cake, and add a little at a time so that it does not get so thick that it cannot be mixed thoroughly. Warn the painter *not* to put water into it because the water would make streaks and paint would peal off the wall.

H.   The class should have a demonstration of the "crawly feeling" explained in Chapter 26, on P page 258 or H page 230. Have ready some pure, untreated cotton, washed with a little baking soda, a piece of carpeting containing a lot of formaldehyde, and a piece of polyester. Have class members use the method suggested on P pages 258–259 or H pages 230–231. With their eyes closed, have them move from one to another, each for thirty seconds, resting a hand lightly on one and then on another—untreated cotton first, polyester second, and carpeting third. Alert them to the differences in sensation. Then have them rub their hands together for a little while. Following that, they should relax their hand and then put it back on the cotton. About fifty percent of the people can be trained to pick up the "crawly feeling" (some people call it a "hot feeling," others call it a "tingling feeling"). Everybody has a different kind of reaction, but will recognize the difference.

For those who may be sensitive to cotton, have available a piece of pure raw silk that has been washed with pure baking soda. Although the sources in the chapter will list Thai and Indian clothes, you must be cautious because many foreign manufacturers are now using toxic fixatives. Sometimes they use ordinary kerosene to fix the dyes of the silk. Therefore, even though the silk may be pure, the dyes are so toxic that they may cause a problem.

Even if patients do not plan on buying or making clothes now, encourage them to read this chapter because, in between the sources, they will find little hints that will be helpful.

The same types of suggestions apply for Chapter 27, which covers home furnishings.

I. In the section "Saving Money" in Class Two, we suggested using items already in the kitchen, such as cucumbers as an astringent. Ask if any students, after reading this material and Chapter 28 in *Coping With Your Allergies*, have found ways to make inexpensive cosmetics. Ask if anyone has other ideas. To reinforce their motivation to search for cost-free methods, you can inform the class that the recipes for cosmetics are included for people who enjoy creating things. The busy mother or career woman can read the recipe, select the important ingredients and use it alone. Cite as an example, the avocado mask. After eating an avocado, using the inside of the skin, the patient can rub the residue on her freshly-scrubbed face and neck. She should leave it on for thirty minutes, while doing some chores, then rinse with warm and then cool water. Voila! A mask, no wasted time, effort, or expense! Remind the class how much money they can save just by giving up perfumes and perfumed products. This is particularly true with cosmetics.

Caution the class, if they own the hardcover copy of *Coping With Your Allergies*, to cross out the reference to Amino Pon Shampoo because it is no longer safe. If they do buy any shampoo, they must check the label to see if it contains formaldehyde.

J. In Chapter 29, "Travel," there are suggestions even for the individual who is not severely sensitive. For example, no one should sit in a parked car for any length of time with the motor running, because the fumes from under the car enter the car. The driver should always leave enough space between his car and the one ahead so that he can inch up slowly.

No one should ever walk behind a car with a running motor. In addition to the danger of the driver suddenly backing up, it is unwise for anyone to have his clothes drenched with the fumes escaping from the tailpipe. We know that the fumes do not easily dissipate because extremely sensitive people can detect those fumes on their clothes hours after such exposure.

III. *The Yeast Connection*, by William P. Crook, M.D. *Note:* Although we have expressed caution in the class material about *The Yeast Connection*, and although Dr. Crook in his book cites the same precautions, it is necessary for you to emphasize more than once during your discussion that this is a very individual problem. This is one situation which *must* be given individual attention under the closest supervision of the doctor.

A. Lead a brief discussion on the chart entitled "Are Your Health Problems Yeast-Connected?" on H page x. To facilitate their study of the subject, illustrate how *The Yeast Connection* has been included in the "Cross-References" section of this book.

B. Discuss the chart called "The Yeast Connection ... A Vicious Cycle" on H page xvi. While the vicious cycle may appear obvious, it is important to point out exactly how it works. Have the class members follow the boxes and arrows, reading aloud.

1. The broad-spectrum antibiotics kill good germs along with the bad. Birth control pills, cortisone, and other drugs, as well as diets rich in yeast and carbohydrates, especially sugar, also cause the yeast to multiply. The multiplication of yeast causes toxins that adversely affect the immune system.

2. The immune system is adversely affected also by

nutritional deficiencies, heavy chemical exposure and heavy mold exposure.

3. When your immune system is adversely affected, your resistance is lessened, which leads you to develop nervous system, digestive, respiratory, and other symptoms.

4. When your resistance is lessened, you also react adversely to things you eat, breathe and touch. Your membranes (nose, throat, bladder, etc.) swell, you develop infections which put you back on broad-spectrum antibiotics, which completes the vicious cycle.

C. Turn to the drawing on page 8 and demonstrate that there are attacker cells and defender cells, and that the defender cells protect you against the attacker cells.

D. Looking at the drawing page 10: highlight the normal intestinal tract and vagina and the ratio of friendly germs, yeast germs, and enemies. Contrast it with the drawing on page 11, which shows the weakened immune system, in which the yeasts multiply and in which there is a changed ratio with a preponderance of yeast germs and the introduction of toxins.

E. Ask the class how many have completed the Candida Questionnaire and Score Sheet on pages 29–33. Lead a brief discussion and encourage the exchange of personal insights among the patients.

F. Referring to Chapter 7, discuss how to treat the Candida problem. Show how diet is one thing that a person can do on his own. Refer the class back to *If This Is Tuesday, It Must Be Chicken* and illustrate how they can follow the diet totally, rotating their foods. When they consult with the physician, the physician can then determine if they have to restrict the unrefined carbohydrates.

Refer the yeast-sensitive patient to the Bibliography for books that teach him to recognize low-carbohydrate foods.

G. By using the formula on page 14 of *If This Is Tuesday, It Must Be Chicken*, tell them that they can use any of the yeast-free recipes without breaking their rotation, unless the recipe calls for a food they must avoid, or a packaged food with multiple ingredients.

Because many of the recipes include herbs and teas, caution the mold-sensitive patient to use those that are fresh or home frozen.

H. For additional information about yeast, malt, and molds, refer them to appendix B15 in *Allergies and the Hyperactive Child* and chapter 11 *Coping with Your Allergies.*

IV. Remember these procedures:

A. Ask the class if they are having any difficulties with the assigned readings.

B. Ask the class if they have any questions from the previous class.

C. Discuss Assignment for Class Six.

1. Mention that *The Type 1/Type 2 Allergy Relief Program,* while it covers many of the aspects of the other books, introduces a new approach—that of dividing allergies into two types, those that are recognized by conventional allergists and those that comprise the specialty of environmental medicine.

2. Ask the class to turn to section, "Rebuilding Adaptation," in Class Six. Mention the fact that information should not be tried until a later date. It discusses how they can rebuild their adaptation after they have stabilized their environment and their food.

Explain that you understand that they may not know when they will be ready to begin the process of rebuilding their adaptation. If in doubt, they should call for a consultation to discuss the matter.

Lesson Plan for Class Six

I. Discuss the reading assignment in *Type 1/Type 2 Allergy Program.*

    A. Have the class turn to P pages 4–6 or H pages 16 and 17. Direct their attention to type 1 symptoms of the respiratory system. Then turn to P page 6 or H page 18, the respiratory symptoms of type 2. Make a comparison of the cerebral symptoms.

    B. Discuss how the class members can make use of the "From Head to Toe: An Allergy-or-Not Checklist," P pages 17–20 or H pages 29–32. Highlight two or three comparisons, e.g., "Nose," "Breasts," and Back." Emphasize that not all symptoms are allergy. Discuss the importance of recognizing those differences so they will know when to take necessary precautions and consult their doctor.

    C. State that P pages 21–24 or H pages 32–36 are self-explanatory. Point out that it would be important for them to know whether they are type 1, type 2, or both.

    D. Ask if there are any questions. Keep the discussion brief and general. When a personal problem is raised, suggest a private consultation.

II. Special attention might be given to the sections, "Coping With Unavoidable Daily Exposures" (Class Five) and "Rebuilding Adaptation" (Class Six).

    A. Ask if patients have discovered new coping techniques since the course was started.

    B. Advise the class that the Rebuilding Adaptation process was designed for the extremely sensitive. However, after testing is completed and they have reached a state of relative freedom from symptoms, class members can adopt some of the measures to suit their own needs.

III. Emphasize the importance of Chapter 30, "Mental Attitude," in *Coping With Your Allergies.*

IV. Try to bring together all the important aspects of each Class in the course.

A. This can be done by dividing the group into six smaller groups or individuals. Each group or individual can take the lead in summarizing one of the Classes. Tell the summarizers to use the **Bold Side Headings** as a guide through each Class. In this way you can judge the progress the group is making and not spend too much time on any one point.

B. As the work of each Class is reviewed, you can remind the groups of the following:

1. The importance of a positive mental attitude;

2. No one can be a 100 percenter;

3. By just removing one thing from their environment or one food from their diet, many people have found enough of an incentive to go and do more.

C. This is a good time to lead a discussion on what steps class members have taken and how they have benefited from certain precautions they have taken.

D. Tell the class that frequently patients report that family members who felt they had only minor complaints noticed that these complaints disappeared following environmental improvement in the house. As an example, this has proven true with removal of aerosol cans and toxic cleaning products.

E. Acknowledge that you couldn't possibly have covered everything in class. That is the purpose of their owning a certain number of books and of their having this textbook to guide them through all of the extra reading. Let them know that no one expects them to finish all of the reading within the first month or two. Motivate them to study on their own because the more they educate themselves, the more they themselves will understand and be able to convince their families to cooperate.

V. Point out other features found at the back of the textbook.

A. Show how the Bibliography contains descriptive remarks for each book.

B. Tell them to see "Fact Sheets" on formaldehyde, alcohol, phenol, use of tri alkali salts, and enemas.

C. Discuss how the cross-references can be used.

VI. Discuss the HEAL application which follows the Bibliography for the book. Emphasize the importance of having a local support group. Patients can help one another find local sources. Patients can provide support for one another, especially when they cannot talk to their doctor.

A. Support group members share information they have read. They should not automatically do everything that a friend has done, but they may learn of new techniques or procedures to bring to the attention of their doctor.

Clinical ecologists teach their parents to be relatively independent in their health care. Once they are on their own, seeing the doctor no more than once or twice a year, patients need a support group to keep abreast of new developments.

Patients find that some of the people they meet will be friendly not only during the period of recovery but for many years. As the families get together, a cooperative spouse very often can convince a less cooperative spouse how much it has helped to work with rather than fight the program.

B. Make a plea for joining national HEAL. First of all, membership dues give HEAL the power to do battle for patients. In addition, the national HEAL publication provides current nationwide environmental medicine information. HEAL members have been able to use the newsletter for printing various requests. For example, when traveling in another state, they can ask for help in locating organic food, spring water, an all-electric motel, or an environmentally-clean home.

A Final Word to the Counselor

This can be the most productive part for you. For your first few classes, it may be helpful to tape record this segment.

Lead a discussion with the members, covering the following points.

1   Should the classes be lengthened?

2   Was there anything omitted that they wanted included?

3   Is there any constructive criticism for how to improve the class?

4   Should the classes be scheduled further apart or even closer together?

5   What segments did they find most helpful?

It does not have to be in that order. They may wish to bring up other questions. Just remember that it is most important to end the discussion on a positive note.

List of Cross-References

To coordinate the material in the books for the course, we have prepared a list of cross-references. It is organized alphabetically by subject and indicates where the material is located in each book. The listing is not meant to duplicate the index of the books and therefore does not list every reference for every word or subject. Rather, the books and page numbers indicate that the material is dealt with substantively—i.e., it increases knowledge of that particular material.

The course was designed to present a consensus of opinion of leaders in environmental medicine. As you read the books, however, you will find differing opinions on some subjects. As in all other medical disciplines, you will find that there is controversy. Clinical ecology differs from other disciplines by the way it is practiced (encouraging questions from patients). It is important for you to understand differing methods and approaches so that you can discuss them intelligently with your doctor.

To save space, the book titles are not completely written out each time they appear. Instead, a shortened version of each title is used. Following is a listing of the books included, along with the shortened version of their titles as they appear in the cross-reference list:

An Alternative Approach to Allergies by Theron G. Randolph, M.D. and Ralph W. Moss, Ph.D. Appears in the cross-reference list as *Alternative Approach*. (Paperback = P)

or

An Alternative Approach to Allergies by Theron G. Randolph, M.D. and Ralph W. Moss, Ph.D. Appears in the cross-reference list as *Alternative Approach*. (Hardcover Edition = H)

Allergies and the Hyperactive Child by Doris J. Rapp, M.D. Appears in the cross-reference list as *Hyperactive Child*. (Paperback = P)

Coping with Your Allergies by Natalie Golos and Frances Golos Golbitz. The new and updated version. Appears in the cross-reference list as *Coping*. (Paperback = P)

or

Coping with Your Allergies by Natalie Golos and Frances Golos Golbitz. Appears in the cross-reference list as *Coping*. (Hardcover Edition = H)

If This Is Tuesday, It Must Be Chicken by Natalie Golos and Frances Golos Golbitz. Appears in the cross-reference list as *Tuesday*. (Paperback = P)

The Type 1/Type 2 Allergy Relief Program by Alan S. Levin, M.D. and Merla Zellerbach. Appears in the cross-reference list as *Type 1/Type 2*. (Paperback = P)

or

The Type 1/Type 2 Allergy Relief Program by Alan S. Levin, M.D. and Merla Zellerbach. Appears in the cross-reference list as *Type 1/Type 2*. (Hardcover Edition = H)

The Yeast Connection by William G. Crook, M.D. Appears in the cross-reference list as *Yeast*. (Paperback = P)

or

The Yeast Connection by William G. Crook, M.D. Appears in the cross-reference list as *Yeast*. (Hardcover Edition = H)

Addiction and Masked Allergy

ADDICTION
Alternative Approach P 20–28, 36–48; H 16–23, 29– 39
Coping P 31–33, 34–35, 84–85; H 28–30, 31, 76–77
Type 1/Type 2 P 8, 87–90; H 20, 97–99

ADDICTION PYRAMID
Alternative Approach P 22; H 18

MASKED SENSITIVITY
Coping P 31–32, 33, 85; H 28, 30, 77

Biological Food Families

BIOLOGICAL FOOD FAMILY LISTS
Alternative Approach P 263–279; H 223–238
Coping P 108–126; H 99–116
Tuesday P 100–117
Type 1/Type 2 P 187–194; H 193–200

Candida Albicans

See "Yeasts and Molds"

Chemical Sensitivities

GENERAL
Chemicals In Our Food
Alternative Approach P 60–77; H 49–63
Factors Precipitating
Coping P 9–11; H 9–11
How Chemicals Cause Illness
Yeast P 147, 150–151; H 153, 156–157

DIAGNOSIS
Chemical Questionnaire—Randolph
Alternative Approach P 223–236; H 188–200
Detecting Chemical Sensitivities
Coping P 169–178; H 155–163
Simple Tests for Chemical Sensitivities
Hyperactive Child P 192–194

IMMUNOTOXIC CHEMICALS
Four Main Categories
Type 1/Type 2 P 64–65; H 73–74
Seven Top Offenders—Saifer
Type 1/Type 2 P 65–66; H 75

TREATMENT
Alternative Approach P 237–249; H 201–211
Yeast P 147–149; H 153–155

TROUBLEMAKERS AT HOME AND AT WORK
Coping P 48–53; H 44–48

Clinical Ecology

CLINICAL ECOLOGY UNITS (HOSPITAL)
Alternative Approach P 200–211, 280–281; H 168–177, 239–240
Coping P 35; H 32
Type 1/Type 2 P 80–84; H 89–93

CLINICAL ECOLOGY VS. CONVENTIONAL MEDICINE
Alternative Approach P 253–262; H 215–222
Coping P 33; H 30

SOURCES OF FURTHER INFORMATION ON
Alternative Approach P 282–283; H 241–242
Coping P 331–334; H 375–376
Hyperactive Child P 173–176

Clothing and Fabrics

BUYING TIPS
Coping P 261–262, 268–273; H 233–234, 241–246

CHOOSING CLOTHING AND FABRICS
Coping P 189, 194–194, 256–273; H 172, 177–178, 229–246

CLEANING CLOTHING DURING TESTING
Coping P 182; H 166–167

CLEANING CLOTHING IN GENERAL, TIPS FOR
Coping P 233–235; H 212–213

CLOTHING TO USE DURING TESTING
Coping P 173–174; H 158–159

DYES FOR FABRICS
Coping P 265; H 238

SEWING TIPS
Coping P 266–268; H 239–241

SOURCES
Coping P 256–273; H 229–246
Type 1/Type 2 P 198, 202–205, 210; H 203, 207–210, 214

Definitions

ADDICTIVE REACTIONS
Type 1/Type 2 P 87–90; H 97–99

ADDITIVE
Type 1/Type 2 P 179; H 187

ALLERGEN
Type 1/Type 2 P 9, 31–32, 62–68, 179; H 21, 42–44, 71–77, 187

ALLERGIC RHINITIS
Type 1/Type 2 P 179; H 187

ALLERGY
Alternative Approach P 22; H 17
Coping P 30–31; H 27–28
Type 1/Type 2 P 4, 7, 179; H 16, 19, 187

ALLERGY VS. SENSITIVITY
Coping P 30–31; H 27–28

ANAPHYLACTIC SHOCK
Type 1/Type 2 P 179; H 187

ANGIOEDEMA
Type 1/Type 2 P 179; H 187

ANTIBODY
Coping P 30–31; H 27
Type 1/Type 2 P 9, 179; H 21, 187

ANTIGEN
Coping P 30–31; H 27
Type 1/Type 2 P 9, 180; H 21, 187

ANTIHISTAMINE
Type 1/Type 2 P 180; H 187

ASTHMA
Type 1/Type 2 P 180; H 187

CANDIDA ALBICANS
Type 1/Type 2 P 180; H 188
Yeast P 2–4; H 2–4

CANDIDIASIS
Type 1/Type 2 P 180; H 188

CHEMICAL SENSITIVITY
Type 1/Type 2 P 63; H 72

CLINICAL ECOLOGY
Coping P 14, 22–23, 39; H 13, 20–21

CONTACT DERMATITIS
Type 1/Type 2 P 181; H 188

CUMULATIVE REACTION
Type 1/Type 2 P 8, 86–90; H 20, 96–97

DESENSITIZATION
Type 1/Type 2 P 181; H 188

ECZEMA
Type 1/Type 2 P 181; H 189

EDEMA
Type 1/Type 2 P 181; H 189

FIXED REACTION
Type 1/Type 2 P 8, 86; H 20, 96

FOOD ADDICTION
Type 1/Type 2 P 181; H 189

FOOD ADDITIVE
Hyperactive Child P 189

HISTAMINE
Type 1/Type 2 P 182; H 189

HOMEOSTASIS
Type 1/Type 2 P 182; H 189

IMMUNE SYSTEM
Type 1/Type 2 P 182; H 189

INHALANT
Type 1/Type 2 P 182; H 189

IRRITANT
Type 1/Type 2 P 182; H 190

OUTGASSING
Type 1/Type 2 P 64, 67; H 73, 76

PREMENSTRUAL SYNDROME (PMS)
Yeast P 180–182; H 187–188

TOLERANCE THRESHOLD
Type 1/Type 2 P 4, 184; H 16, 191

UNIVERSAL REACTOR
Coping P 33; H 30
Type 1/Type 2 P 78–80, 185; H 87–89, 192

URTICARIA
Type 1/Type 2 P 185; H 192

VARIABLE REACTION
Type 1/Type 2 P 8, 87; H 20, 97

WITHDRAWAL
Type 1/Type 2 P 185; H 192

YEASTS AND MOLDS
Yeast P 2–4, 57–58; H 2–4, 55–56

Diets

ELIMINATION DIETS
General
Hyperactive Child P 89–107, 132–135
Type 1/Type 2 P 90–93; H 99–103
Yeast P 81–85, 122–123, 235; H 75–78, 128–129, 243

Specific
5/5 Allergy-Obesity Diet
  Type 1/Type 2 P 114–121; H 123–129
  Basic Food Sensitivity Diet
  Type 1/Type 2 P 93–100; H 103–109
  Candida Albicans Food Sensitivity Diet
  Type 1/Type 2 P 106; H 115
  Yeast P 41–44, 77–119, 235; H 42–43, 72–125, 243
  Citric-Acid-Free Diet
  Hyperactive Child P 162
  Citrus-Free Diet
  Hyperactive Child P 161
  Corn Allergy, Diet To Check For
  Hyperactive Child P 157–160
  Dye or Food-Coloring Allergy, Diet To Check For
  Hyperactive Child P 154–156
  Fasting
  Alternative Approach P 200–203, 208–209; H 168–171, 175
  Coping P 22, 84; H 20, 76
  Feingold Diet
  Hyperactive Child P 166–168
  Rare Food Diet—Dr. Crook
  Hyperactive Child P 171–172
  Vegetarian Food-Sensitivity Diet
  Type 1/Type 2 P 104–105; H 114–115
  Rotary Diversified Diet (RDD)
  Alternative Approach P 212–222; H 178–187
  Coping P 83–107, 137–138; H 75–98, 127–128
  Hyperactive Child P 79–85
  Tuesday P Entire book
  Type 1/Type 2 P 8–9; H 20
  Yeast P 123–124, 236; H 129–130, 243

Elimination Diets

See "Diets"

Fabrics

See "Clothing and Fabrics"

Foods

GENERAL
Are Your Health Problems Due To Foods? Questions To Ask.

Hyperactive Child P 73–74, 125–127
Food Problems That Are Not Allergy
Hyperactive Child P 85–86, 87–88

ADDITIVES
Hyperactive Child P 169–170

ADDITIVE-FREE FOODS—FINDING THEM
Coping P 174–75; H 160

ANTIBIOTICS AND HORMONES IN FOODS
Alternative Approach P 74; H 60–61

CHEMICALS IN FOODS
General
Alternative Approach P 60–77; H 49–63
Hyperactive Child P 189–191

CLOROX RINSE FOR FRUITS AND VEGETABLES
Yeast P 250–251; H 256–257

COLORS AND FLAVORS—ARTIFICIAL
Alternative Approach P 67–68; H 55–56
Hyperactive Child P 8; 154–156

COOKING AND RECIPES
Coping P 137–166, 309–366; H 127–151, 279–326
Hyperactive Child P 136–140
Tuesday Throughout book
Type 1/Type 2 P 100–104; H 109–113
Yeast P 109–114; H 111–117, 123–125

FOODS EXPOSED TO GAS
Alternative Approach P 69–70; H 56–58

OBVIOUS VS. HIDDEN ALLERGIES
Coping P 21–29; H 19–26
Yeast P 122, 235–236; H 128, 243

PACKAGING MATERIALS
Alternative Approach P 71; H 58
Coping P 139–144, 174, 186–188, 367–370; H 129–133, 161, 170–171

PESTICIDE SPRAY, RESIDUES ON FOODS
Alternative Approach P 61–67; H 50–55

RELATIVELY SAFE FOODS
Alternative Approach P 74–75; H 61–62

Coping P 127–131; H 117–120
Hyperactive Child P 191

SUBSTITUTIONS
Coping P 145–147; H 134–142
Tuesday P 124

SUGAR SUBSTITUTES
Yeast P 117–119; H 123–125

SULFUR
Alternative Approach P 66–67; H 54–55

VARIABLE (INTERMITTENT) REACTIONS TO FOODS
Hyperactive Child P 79

WATER
Alternative Approach P 75–77; H 62–63
Coping P 37; H 33
Hyperactive Child P 193–194

WAXES ON FOODS
Alternative Approach P 73–74; H 60

YEAST CONTACT, COMMON SOURCES OF
Hyperactive Child P 164–165

YEASTS AND MOLDS IN FOODS
Coping P 132–134; H 121–123
Yeast P 2–4, 57–58, 115–116; H 2–4, 55–56, 121–123

Health Needs

FIRST AID HINTS AND SUPPLIES
Coping P 197–202; H 179–183

Housing

GENERAL
Coping P 211–226; H 193–205

BEDROOM
Ideal Type 1 Bedroom
Type 1/Type 2 P 128–129; H 136–137

Ideal Type 2 Bedroom
Type 1/Type 2 P 129–131; H 137–138
Making Bedroom Allergen-Free
Alternative Approach P 245–247; H 207–210
Coping P 179–182; H 164–166

FUELS—TYPE THAT SHOULD BE USED
Hyperactive Child P 188

HOME FURNISHINGS
Coping P 274–280; H 247–253

HOME HEATING SYSTEMS
Alternative Approach P 242–243; H 205–206

MAKING HOME ALLERGEN-FREE
Alternative Approach P 237–249; H 201–211
Hyperactive Child P 183–186

PAINT—TYPE THAT SHOULD BE USED
Hyperactive Child P 188

TROUBLEMAKERS IN THE HOME
Coping P 48–53; H 44–48

Human Ecology Action League (HEAL)

GENERAL
Coping P 28–29, 371; H 25–26, 332

Illnesses/Symptoms

GENERAL
Type 1/Type 2 P 4–7; H 16–19
Miscellaneous Medical Problems and Possible Major Food or Other Suspects
Hyperactive Child P 126–127
From Head To Toe: An Allergy-or-Not checklist
Type 1/Type 2 P 17–20; H 29–32
Possible Symptoms of Allergy in Questionnaire Form
Hyperactive Child P 66–68
Stages And Symptoms of Environmental Disease
Alternative Approach P 115–185; H 97–155

ALCOHOLISM
Alternative Approach P 40, 118–119, 129–138; H 32–33, 100, 109–116

Hyperactive Child P 113–14
Type 1/Type 2 P 109–110; H 118–119

Symptoms of Alcoholism When No Alcohol Has Been Consumed
Yeast P 221–222; H 229–230

ALLERGIC FACE
Hyperactive Child P 60–66

ALLERGIC RHINITIS
Type 1/Type 2 P 26–27; 38–40; H 38, 49–51

ANOREXIA NERVOSA
Hyperactive Child P 114

ARTHRITIS
Alternative Approach P 153–163; H 129–137
Coping P 33–34; H 30–31
Yeast P 215–216; H 223–224

ASTHMA
Alternative Approach P 140–141; H 118
Type 1/Type 2 P 27–28, 40–42; H 38–39, 51–53

BEHAVIORAL/CEREBRAL PROBLEMS
General
Coping P 34–35; H 31
Hyperactive Child P 108–112
Type 1/Type 2 P 30, 55–58; H 42, 64–67
Allergic-Tension-Fatigue Syndrome
Alternative Approach P 143; H 120
Hyperactive Child P 4–7, 12–16
Behavior Ups and Downs
Alternative Approach P 36–48; H 29–39
Brain Fag
Alternative Approach P 43–44, 117, 144, 164–174; H 35–36, 99, 121, 138–146
Depression
Alternative Approach P 144–145, 175–185, 254; H 121–122, 147–155, 216
Coping P 54–61, 301–306; H 49–55, 272–276
Fatigue
Alternative Approach P 143–144, 164–174, 254; H 121, 138–146, 216
Fatigue after Meals
Coping P 37; H 34
Headache
Alternative Approach P 146–152; H 123–128
Type 1/Type 2 P 58–62, H 67–71
Hyperactivity

Alternative Approach P 120–128; H 101–108
Coping P 22; H 20
Hyperactive Child P 8, 9–12, 23–59
Hyperactivity—Relationship to Allergy
Hyperactive Child P 3–22
Mental Illness
Alternative Approach P 8–9, 38–48, 115–119, 139–145, 164, 167–168, 175–177, 254–258; H 6–7, 29–39, 97–100, 117–122, 138, 140–141, 147–148, 216–219
Coping P 54–61; H 49–55
Mental Retardation
Hyperactive Child P 115–117
Migraine Headaches
Alternative Approach P 142–143, 146–152; H 120, 123–128
Coping P 31; H 27
Type 1/Type 2 P 58–62; H 67–71
Minimal Brain Dysfunction (MBD)
Hyperactive Child P 7–8, 26–28
Specific Learning Disability (SLD)
Hyperactive Child P 26

BODY ODOR
Coping P 37–38; H 34

CANDIDA ALBICANS
Type 1/Type 2 P 67–68, 74–76; H 76–77, 83–84
Yeast P Entire book; H Entire book
See Also "Yeasts and Molds"

CARDIOVASCULAR SYMPTOMS
General
Alternative Approach P 42–43, 142; H 34, 119–120

DRUGS AS CAUSE
Alternative Approach P 78–83; H 64–68

GASTROINTESTINAL SYMPTOMS
General
Alternative Approach P 42, 116–117, 141–142; H 34, 98, 119
Type 1/Type 2 P 30; H 42

GENITOURINARY SYSTEM SYMPTOMS
General
Alternative Approach P 116–117, 142; H 98, 119

HEART DISEASE
Coping P 62–66; H 56–59

HIVES
Alternative Approach P 141; H 119
Type 1/Type 2 P 29–30; H 41

HUNGER
Alternative Approach P 39, 118; H 32, 99
Coping P 37; H 33

HYPOGLYCEMIA
Hyperactive Child P 55–59

INFERTILITY
Hyperactive Child P 114

INSECT BITE TREATMENTS AS CAUSE
Type 1/Type 2 P 45; H 56

MISCELLANEOUS MEDICAL PROBLEMS AND POSSIBLE MAJOR FOOD OR OTHER
SUSPECTS
Hyperactive Child P 126–127

MULTIPLE SCLEROSIS (MS)
Yeast P 223–231; H 218–227

OBESITY
Alternative Approach P 39, 118–119; H 32, 99, 100
Hyperactive Child P 114
Type 1/Type 2 P 110–114; H 119–123

RESPIRATORY SYMPTOMS
General
Alternative Approach P 42, 116, 140–141; H 34, 98, 118

SEIZURES
Hyperactive Child P 114–15

SEXUAL PROBLEMS
Hyperactive Child P 114

SKIN DISORDERS
General
Alternative Approach P 141; H 118–119
Type 1/Type 2 P 28–30; H 40–41
Eczema
Type 1/Type 2 P 28–30, 44–45; H 40–42, 54–55
Hives

Type 1/Type 2 P 29–30; H 41
Insect Bites and Stings
Type 1/Type 2 P 30; H 41–42
Poison Ivy And Poison Oak
Type 1/Type 2 P 28; H 40

SPEECH PROBLEMS
Hyperactive Child P 114

SUICIDE
Hyperactive Child P 115

TEMPERATURE (HEAT AND COLD) SENSITIVITY
Type 1/Type 2 P 31–32; H 42–44

TYPE 1 SYMPTOMS
General
Type 1/Type 2 P 4–6, 26–30; H 16–17, 38–42

TYPE 2 SYMPTOMS
General
Type 1/Type 2 P 6–7, 55–62; H 18–19, 67–71

WITHDRAWAL LEVELS OF REACTION
Alternative Approach P 139–145; H 117–122

Immune System

GENERAL
How It Works
Yeast P 8–15, 137, 157–160; H 8–15, 143, 163–166
Immune System Regulation
  IgE
  Type 1/Type 2 P 11–13; H 23–24
  T-Cells and B-Cells
  Type 1/Type 2 P 11–13; H 23–24

Indoor Pollution

GENERAL
Alternative Approach P 84–101; H 69–83
Hyperactive Child P 188–191
Type 1/Type 2 P 64–67; H 73–76

ADHESIVES
Hyperactive Child P 188

ALCOHOL
Hyperactive Child P 188

ALUMINUM
Coping P 51, 175, 188; H 46, 160–161, 172
Yeast P 133; H 139

AUTOMOBILES
Alternative Approach P 94–96, 243–245; H 78–79, 206–207
Coping P 51, 195–196; H 46

CHEMICALS, IMMUNOTOXIC
Coping P 48–53, 169–178; H 44–48, 155–163
Type 1/Type 2 P 62–63; H 72

CIGARETTES
Alternative Approach P 141, 240–241; H 118, 203–204

CIGARETTE SMOKE
Coping P 38–39, 52; H 34–35, 47

CLEANING FLUIDS AND LIGHTER FLUIDS
Alternative Approach P 90–91, 96, 98–101, 241–242; H 74–75, 79, 81–83, 204–205
Hyperactive Child P 188

DETERGENTS AND SOAPS
Alternative Approach P 96, 98–101, 241–242; H 79, 81–83, 204–205
Coping P 51–52, 56–57, 189–192, 227–235, 288, 367–370; H 47, 52–53, 173–175, 206–213, 260

ELECTROMAGNETIC POLLUTION
Coping P 27–28 (Not in hardcover)

FORMALDEHYDE
Alternative Approach P 58–59, 97, 140; H 48, 80, 129–130
Coping P 52 (Not in hardcover)

FUELS
Alternative Approach P 85–89; H 70–73
Hyperactive Child P 188

INSECTICIDES
Hyperactive Child P 188

Yeast P 53–54, 57–59; H 52, 55–57

MECHANICAL DEVICES AND MOTORS
Alternative Approach P 94; H 77–78
Coping P 141; H 131
Hyperactive Child P 189

MISCELLANEOUS MEDICAL PROBLEMS AND POSSIBLE MAJOR FOOD OR OTHER SUSPECTS
Hyperactive Child P 126–127

MOLDS
Coping P 143, 213–214, 216, 217, 223, 234–235, 278; H 133, 195, 198, 203, 209–210, 213, 251
Yeast P 53–54, 57–59; H 52, 55–57

NEWSPRINT
Hyperactive Child P 188

OFFICE, COMMON CONTAMINANTS IN
Type 1/Type 2 P 135–139; H 142–147

OUTGASSING
Type 1/Type 2 P 64, 67; H 73, 76

OUTGASSING CAPACITY OF COMMON MATERIALS
Type 1/Type 2 P 65–67; H 74–76

PERFUMES
Alternative Approach P 82–83; H 68

PESTICIDES
Alternative Approach P 61–66, 91–92, 109–112; H 50– 54, 75–76, 90–93
Coping P 27, 51, 170, 231; H 24–25, 47, 155–156, 210

PETROLEUM PRODUCTS
Coping P 170; H 156
Yeast P 146–147; H 152–153

PLASTICS
Alternative Approach P 93–94; H 77
Coping P 49, 170–171, 186–188; H 45, 156, 170–71
Hyperactive Child P 189

REFRIGERANTS
Alternative Approach P 91; H 75

Coping P 52, 222–223; H 47, 202
Hyperactive Child P 188

SCHOOLS, POLLUTANTS IN
Hyperactive Child P 70–71

SOLVENTS (PAINT, VARNISH, ETC.)
Alternative Approach P 89–90; H 73–74
Coping P 52, 171; H 47, 156–157

SPONGE RUBBER
Alternative Approach P 93; H 76–77
Coping P 52; H 47
Hyperactive Child P 189

SPRAY CONTAINERS
Alternative Approach P 91; H 75
Coping P 51; H 46
Hyperactive Child P 188

TROUBLEMAKERS AT HOME AND AT WORK
Coping P 48–53; H 44–48
Type 1/Type 2 P 135–139; H 142–147

YEASTS AND MOLDS
Defined
Yeast P 2–4, 58–59; H 2–4; 55–56
See "Yeasts and Molds"

Mental Attitude

POSITIVE MENTAL ATTITUDE, IMPORTANCE OF
Coping P 301–306; H 272–276

STRESS
Coping P 33; H 29–30

STRESS REDUCTION
Coping P 67–80; H 60–72
Type 1/Type 2 P 163; H 171

Miscellaneous

AIR IONIZERS
Yeast P 249; H 255

AIR PURIFIERS
Type 1/Type 2 P 129; H 137

ASSOCIATIONS AND THEIR PUBLICATIONS
Coping P 371–373 (Not in hardcover)

CLEANING TIPS AND AIDS
Coping P 227–235; H 206–213

DENTAL CARE
Coping P 189 (Not in hardcover)

EXERCISE
Coping P 303; H 273–275
Type 1/Type 2 P 166–167; H 174–175

FIRST AID HINTS AND SUPPLIES
Coping P 197–202; H 179–183

HORMONE IMBALANCE
Yeast P 244–245; H 251–252

ILLNESS, CAUSES OF
General
Yeast P 138–141; H 144–147

LACTOSE INTOLERANCE
Hyperactive Child P 31–32

MEDICAL PRACTITIONER
Choosing a Doctor
Type 1/Type 2 P 145–152; H 152–159
Educating the Medical Practitioner
Coping P 203–208; H 184–189

NEWSPRINT, RECOMMENDATIONS FOR HANDLING
General
Hyperactive Child P 188
Reading Box
Coping P 184–186; H 168–169

OBVIOUS VS. HIDDEN ALLERGIES
Coping P 21–29; H 19–26
Yeast P 122, 235; H 128, 243

OPTIMUM HEALTH, FACTORS NECESSARY FOR
General

Yeast P 136–137; H 142–143

PEST CONTROL
Coping P 236–255; H 214–228

POLLEN CALENDAR
Hyperactive Child P 180–182

PREVENTION OF ALLERGIES
Coping P 40–47, 49–53; H 36–43, 45–47

SHOPPING TIPS—MAKING LIFE EASIER
Coping P 193–196; H 176–178

TIPS FOR THE BEGINNER WITH COMPLEX ALLERGIES—HOW TO DETOXIFY HIS/HER
LIFE
Coping P 184–192; H 168–175

TYPE 1 PERSON—PROFILE
Type 1/Type 2 P 3–4, 25–51, 184; H 14–16, 37–62, 191

TYPE 2 PERSON—PROFILE
Type 1/Type 2 P 3–4, 53–84, 184–185; H 14–16, 63–93, 191

Nutritional Information

GENERAL
Yeast P 131–133; H 137–139

NUTRIENTS, DEPLETION OF BY SUGAR
Coping P 309–310; H 279

Outdoor Pollution

GENERAL
Alternative Approach P 102–112; H 84–93
Type 1/Type 2 P 64–66; H 73–75

CIGARETTES
Alternative Approach P 141, 240–241; H 118, 203–204
Coping P 38–39; H 34–35

CHEMICALS—IMMUNOTOXIC
Coping P 48–53; 169–178; H 44–48, 155–163

Type 1/Type 2 P 62–63; H 72

ELECTROMAGNETIC POLLUTION
Coping P 62–63; H 72

FOGGING FOR INSECT ABATEMENT
Alternative Approach P 109–110; H 90–93

FORMALDEHYDE
Alternative Approach P 97; H 80
Coping P 52 (Not in hardcover)

FUELS
Alternative Approach P 85–89; H 70–73

INSECTICIDES
Yeast P 133; H 139

LEAD
Yeast P 133; H 139

MECHANICAL DEVICES AND MOTORS
Alternative Approach P 94; H 77–78
Coping P 141; H 131

MISCELLANEOUS MEDICAL PROBLEMS AND POSSIBLE MAJOR FOOD OR OTHER
SUSPECTS
Hyperactive Child P 126–127

OUTGASSING
Type 1/Type 2 P 64–67; H 73, 76

OUTGASSING CAPACITY OF COMMON MATERIALS
Type 1/Type 2 P 65–67; H 74–76

PETROLEUM PRODUCTS
Coping P 170; H 156
Yeast P 146–147; H 152–153

PLASTICS
Alternative Approach P 93–94; H 77

SOLVENTS (PAINT, VARNISH, ETC.)
Alternative Approach P 89–90; H 73–74

VEHICLE EXHAUST
Alternative Approach P 104–109; H 86–90

YEAST AND MOLDS
See "Yeasts and Molds"

Personal Hygiene

COSMETICS AND PERSONAL HYGIENE ITEMS
Alternative Approach P 82–83; H 68
Coping P 186–192, 281–288; H 170–175, 254–260

DEODORANT, NATURAL
Coping P 38; H 34

Product Sources

TYPES, BRANDS AND COMPANIES
General
Coping P 367–370 (Not in hardcover)
Type 1/Type 2 P 197–210; H 203–214

Specific
  Adhesive Bandages
  Coping P 188; H 171
  Air Filters
  Type 1/Type 2 P 197; H 203
  Anesthetics
  Coping P 188; H 171
  Cellophane Food Wrap
  Type 1/Type 2 P 202; H 207
  Cleaning Aids
  Coping P 227–235, 367–370; H 206–213
  Clothing And Fabrics
  Coping P 256–273, 367–370; H 229–246
  Type 1/Type 2 P 198, 202–205, 210; H 203, 207–210, 214
  Cosmetics and Toiletries
  Coping P 281–288, 367–370; H 254–260
  Type 1/Type 2 P 198; H 203–204
  Feminine Protection
  Type 1/Type 2 P 205; H 210
  Food
    General
    Type 1/Type 2 P 206–207; H 211–212
    Relatively Safe Food From Commercial Sources
    Coping P 127–131, 367–370; H 117–120
  Glues
  Coping P 119, 225; H 173, 204

Heaters
Coping P 181–182, 218–219; H 166, 200
Home Furnishings
Coping P 274–280, 367–370; H 247–253
Type 1/Type 2 P 198–201, 208; H 204–207, 212–213
Housing Materials
  General
  Coping P 211–226, 367–370; H 193–205
  Kitchen Appliances
  Coping P 140, 159, 215, 221, 222–223, 224; H 129, 144, 196–197, 201, 202, 203
  Kitchen Utensils
  Coping P 139, 158–159, 175, 186–187, 367–370; H 129–143, 144, 160–161, 170–171
Motor Oils
Coping P 191, 292; H 174, 264
Pens
Coping P 186; H 170
Pest Control Materials
Coping P 236–255; H 214–228
Reading Box
Coping P 184–186; H 168
Type 1/Type 2 P 207; H 212
Travel Materials
Coping P 289–300; H 261–271
Water Filters
Type 1/Type 2 P 209; H 214

Rotary Diversified Diet (RDD)

See "Diets"

Supplements

Alternative Approach P 79–81; 221–222; H 65–66, 186
Hyperactive Child P 47–55
Type 1/Type 2 P 167–168; H 175–176
Yeast P 132, 236–240; H 138, 243–246

Testing/Diagnosis

ARE YOUR HEALTH PROBLEMS DUE TO A FOOD? QUESTIONS TO ASK.
Hyperactive Child P 73–74

ALLERGY SMEAR
Type 1/Type 2 P 35; H 46

AVOIDANCE AND CHALLENGE
Coping P 35–36; H 32
Type 1/Type 2 P 36–37; H 47–48

CHEMICAL QUESTIONNAIRE—RANDOLPH
Alternative Approach P 223–236; H 188–200

CYTOTOXIC TEST
Type 1/Type 2 P 70; H 79–80

DIETS
See "Diets"

FABRICS, TEST FOR
Coping P 258–260; H 230–232

INTRADERMAL TESTS
Type 1/Type 2 P 33, 182; H 44, 190

MEDICAL HISTORY
Alternative Approach P 192–195; H 161–163

PROVOCATIVE NEUTRALIZATION (P-N)
Type 1/Type 2 P 10, 11, 183; H 22, 23, 190

PROVOCATIVE NEUTRALIZATION (P-N) INTRADERMAL TEST
Coping P 36–37; H 33
Hyperactive Child P 101
Type 1/Type 2 P 33–34; H 45

PROVOCATIVE/NEUTRALIZATION (P-N) SUBLINGUAL TEST
Alternative Approach P 195–199; H 163–167
Coping P 36; H 32–33
Hyperactive Child P 101
Type 1/Type 2 P 71–72; H 80–81

PULSE TEST
Type 1/Type 2 P 37, 183; H 48, 191

RAST TEST
Type 1/Type 2 P 34–35; H 45–46

SCRATCH TESTS
Coping P 35; H 27, 32
Type 1/Type 2 P 9–10, 33; H 21, 44

SIMPLE TESTS FOR CHEMICAL SENSITIVITIES
Hyperactive Child P 192–194

SNIFF TEST
Coping P 260; H 232
Type 1/Type 2 P 69–70; H 78–79

T AND B BLOOD CELL COUNT AND HELPER/SUPPRESSOR RATIOS

T-CELL SUBSETS
Type 1/Type 2 P 70; H 79

TESTING FOR COMPLEX ALLERGIES AT HOME
Coping P 169–178; H 155–163

TEST TO DETERMINE WHETHER YOU ARE A TYPE 1 OR TYPE 2
Type 1/Type 2 P 21–27; H 32–36

Travel

TRAVEL REQUIREMENTS
Coping P 289–300; H 261–270
Type 1/Type 2 P 139–145; H 147–152

Treatment

GENERAL
Alternative Approach P 189–249; H 159–211

ALKALI SALTS
Coping P 198; H 180
Hyperactive Child P 76
Type 1/Type 2 P 69; H 78

ALLERGIC RHINITIS (HAY FEVER), TREATMENTS FOR
Type 1/Type 2 P 38–40; H 49–51

ASTHMA—TREATMENTS FOR
Type 1/Type 2 P 40–42; H 51–53

CLEANING TIPS AND AIDS
Coping P 227–235; H 206–213

EXERCISE
Coping P 303–304; H 273–275
Type 1/Type 2 P 166–167; H 174–175

FIRST AID HINTS AND SUPPLIES
Coping P 197–202; H 179–183

DESENSITIZING SHOTS
Type 1/Type 2 P 10; H 21–22

IMMUNOTHERAPY
Yeast P 246–249; H 252–255

INSECT STINGS AND BITES, TREATMENTS FOR
Type 1/Type 2 P 45; H 55–56

MEDICATIONS FOR TYPE 1
Type 1/Type 2 P 47–51; H 57–61

PEST CONTROL
Coping P 236–255; H 214–228

POSITIVE MENTAL ATTITUDE
Coping P 301–306; H 272–276

PROVOCATIVE NEUTRALIZATION (P-N)
Type 1/Type 2 P 10, 11; H 22, 23

READING BOX
Coping P 184–186; H 168–169

ROTARY DIVERSIFIED DIET (RDD)
See "Diets"

SKIN DISORDERS, TREATMENT FOR
Type 1/Type 2 P 42–45; H 53–55

STRESS REDUCTION
Coping P 67–80; H 60–72
Type 1/Type 2 P 163; H 171

SUBLINGUAL ANTIGENS FOR ALLERGIC RHINITIS (HAY FEVER)
Type 1/Type 2 P 38–40; H 49–50

SUPPLEMENTS
Alternative Approach P 79–81, 221–222; H 65–66, 186

Type 1/Type 2 P 167–168; H 175–176
Yeast P 132–133, 236–240; H 138, 243–246

TEMPERATURE (HEAT AND COLD) SENSITIVITY-TREATMENTS FOR
Type 1/Type 2 P 45–56; H 56–57

Yeasts and Molds

DEFINED
Coping P 132–134; H 121–123
Yeast P 2–4, 57–58; H 2–4; 55–56

CANDIDA ALBICANS
General
Coping P 134 (Not in hardcover)
Type 1/Type 2 P 67–68; H 76–77
Causes of Health Problems from
Coping P 134 (Not in hardcover)
Yeast P 14, 15, 17–26; H 14, 15, 17–26
Antibiotics As A Cause of Problems From
Coping P 134 (Not in hardcover)
Yeast P 11–12, 14; H xi, 11–12, 14
Candida Albicans Defined
Coping P 134 (Not in hardcover)
Type 1/Type 2 P 180; H 188
Yeast P 2–4; H 2–4
Candidiasis Defined
Type 1/Type 2 P 180; H 188
Yeasts and Molds Defined
Yeast P 2–4, 57–58; H 2–4, 55–56
Diagnosis of Problems with Candida Albicans
Yeast P 27–28, 29–33, 40; H 27–28, 29–33, 40
Immune System and Candida Albicans
How the Immune System Works
Yeast P 8–15, 137, 157–160; H 8–15, 143, 163–166
Yeasts Effect on the Immune System
Coping P 134; (Not in hardcover)
Yeast P 8–15; H xi–xii, 8–15
Medications for the Treatment of Candida Albicans
Amphotericin B
  Yeast P 53, 281–285; H 51, 279–282
  Cloterimazole
  Yeast P 250; H 256
  Ketoconazole (Nizoral)
  Yeast P 49–53; H 48–51
  Nystatin (Nilstat, Mycostatin)

Type 1/Type 2 P 74–76; H 83–84
Yeast P 45–49, 240–242; H 44–50, 247–249
Miscellaneous
  Clorox Rinse for Fruits and Vegetables
  Yeast P 250–251; H 256–257
  Summary of the 1982 Dallas Informal Conference re. Candida Albicans
  Yeast P 270–272; H 261–265
Molds and Candida Albicans
  Sources of Molds
  Yeast P 58–59; H 51, 56–57
Multiple Sclerosis (MS) and Candida Albicans
Yeast P 210–219; H 218–227
Premenstrual Syndrome (PMS) and Candida Albicans
Yeast P 333–338; H 187–188
Supplements and Candida Albicans
Yeast P 132–133, 230–240, 249; H 138, 243–246, 255
Symptoms (Possible) of Candida Albicans as a Problem
  General
  Coping P 134 (Not in hardcover)
  Yeast P 210–219; H viii, ix–x, 218–227
  In Children
  Yeast P 189–204; H 195–211
  In Men
  Yeast P 185–188; H 191–194
  In Teenagers
  Yeast P 205–209; H 213–217
  In Women
  Yeast P 172–184; H 178–190
  Thrush
  Yeast P 3; H 3
Treatment of Candida Albicans
  General
  Yeast P 35–55, 56–64, 67–124, 234–258; H 35–53, 54–64, 67–175, 243–264
  Diets for
  General
  Type 1/Type 2 P 106; H 115
  Yeast P 41–44, 67–119, 235–236; H 42–43, 72–125, 243
  Sugar Substitutes
  Yeast P 117–119; H 123–125
  Digestive Enzymes and Candida Albicans
  Yeast P 250; H 256
  Immunotherapy
  Yeast P 246–250; H 252–255
  La Pacho Tea (Taheebo Tea)
  Type 1/Type 2 P 76; H 85
  Yeast P 251; H 250–251
  Recipes, Yeast-Free
  Yeast P 109–114; H 111–117

Yeast Vaccine
Yeast P 54, 246–249; H 51, 252–253

CLOROX RINSE FOR FRUITS AND VEGETABLES
Yeast P 250–251; H 256–257

CONTROLLING YEASTS AND MOLDS
Yeast P 59–64; H 57–64

RECIPES, YEAST-FREE
Yeast P 109–114; H 111–117

SOURCES OF CONTACT WITH YEASTS AND MOLDS
Coping P 132–134; H 121–123
Hyperactive Child P 164–165
Yeast P 58–59; H 56–57

SUPPLEMENTS
Yeast P 132–133, 235–239, 249; H 138, 243–246, 255

SYMPTOMS OF YEAST-CONNECTED HEALTH PROBLEMS (POSSIBLE)
General
Coping P 134 (Not in hardcover)
Yeast P 210–219; H viii, ix–x, 218–228
In Children
Yeast P 189–204; H 195–211
In Men
Yeast P 185–188; H 191–194
In Teenagers
Yeast P 205–209; H 213–217
In Women
Yeast P 172–184; H 178–190

Bibliography

The publications in this Bibliography represent a broad overview of the field of clinical ecology. Each book expresses the viewpoint of its author or authors. Its inclusion here is not meant to support or refute all material which it includes. "P" refers to paperback and "H" refers to hardcover.

Bell, Iris R., M.D., Ph.D. *Clinical Ecology.* Bolinas, California: Common Knowledge Press, 1982. (P)
>   A technical overview of clinical ecology by a doctor who practices it. Because it is short and concise, it is a must for the reader with either some technical background or some prior contact with the subject.

Coca, Arthur F., M.D. *The Pulse Test.* New York: Arco Publishing Company, 1978. (P)
>   A look at one way of diagnosing food and chemical allergies.

Crook, William G., M.D. *Are You Allergic?* Jackson, Tennessee: Professional Books, 1974. (P)
>   An overview of allergy for the lay reader.

————. *Tracking Down Hidden Food Allergies.* Jackson, Tennessee: Professional Books, 1978. (P)
>   A concise introduction to food allergies, brought to life by illustrations and simple explanations. Especially appropriate for beginners. An excellent book for parents and their allergic children to read together.

————. *Yeasts And How They Can Make You Sick.* Jackson, Tennessee: Professional Books, 1984. (P).

————. *The Yeast Connection.* Jackson, Tennessee: Professional Books, 1983. (H)
>   In both books, Crook discusses the relationship role of yeast/mold sensitivities with environmental illness.

Dickey, Lawrence D., M.D., ed. *Clinical Ecology.* Springfield, Illinois: Charles C. Thomas, 1976. (H)
>   A technical collection of articles by leaders in the field of clinical ecology, covering many issues in the field, including theories, history, diagnosis, and treatment. A good book for the reader with either medical knowledge or a good deal of prior reading in the field.

Dodd, Debra Lynn, "Nontoxic—Natural: How to Avoid Dangerous Products and Make Healthy Ones." Los Angeles: Tarcher, 1984.

Forman, Robert, Ph.D. *How To Control Your Allergies.* New York: Larchmont Books, 1979. (P)
>   An easy-to-read overview of food and chemical allergies, appropriate for the lay reader.

Gerrard, John W. *Food Allergy.* Springfield, Illinois: Charles C. Thomas, 1980. (P)
> An international consort of experts explains food allergy, its mechanisms, its effects on various organ systems, and its medical management.

Golos, Natalie, and Frances Golos Golbitz. *Coping With Your Allergies.* New York: Simon and Schuster, 1979; Fireside, 1986. (P)
> A comprehensive, practical guide for the patient with food and chemical susceptibility. It includes prevention, treatment for the person who is not totally incapacitated, and treatment for the severely allergic.

————. *If This Is Tuesday, It Must Be Chicken.* New Canaan, Connecticut: Keats Publishing, 1983. (P)
> A practical guide to the rotary diversified diet as it should be used for the prevention, diagnosis, and treatment of food allergies.

Hill, Amelia Nathan. *Against the Unsuspected Enemy.* W. Sussex, England: New Horizon, 1980. (P)
> The personal story of a woman plagued for many years by debilitating ecological illness, but who is finally helped by a clinical ecologist.

Hills, Hilda Cherry. *Good Food, Gluten Free.* New Canaan, Connecticut: Keats Publishing, Inc., 1976. (H)

Hunter, Beatrice Trum. *Beatrice Trum Hunter's Additive Book.* New Canaan, Connecticut: Keats Publishing, Inc., 1980.

————. *Consumer, Beware.* New York: Simon and Schuster, 1971.
> A penetrating analysis of how our food supply has been adulterated and its nutrients lost.

————. *How Safe Is Food in Your Kitchen?* New York: Scribner's, 1981.

Ilg, Frances L., M.D., Louise Bates Ames, Ph.D., and Sidney M. Baker, M.D. *Child Behavior.* New York: Harper & Row, 1981. (H)
> A multi-dimensional approach to child behavior that makes use of clinical ecology. The book comes from the well-known Gesell Institute for Human Behavior.

Levin, Alan Scott, M.D. and Merla Zellerbach. *The Type 1/Type 2 Allergy Relief Program.* Los Angeles: Jeremy P. Tarcher, Inc., 1983. (H)
> An excellent overview which offers insight into different types of treatment for different types of allergies.

Mackarness, Richard M., M.D. *Chemical Victims.* London: Pan Books, 1980. (P)
> A historical approach to ecologic illness, with special emphasis on how chemicals are destructive to physical and mental health.

————. *Not All in the Mind.* London: Pan Books, 1976. (P) Published in the U.S. (H), as *Eating Dangerously*, now out of print.
> An excellent introduction to clinical ecology, with an emphasis on food allergies and the "Stone Age Diet."

Mandell, Marshall, M.D., and Lynne Waller Scanlon. *Dr. Mandell's 5-Day Allergy Relief System.* New York: Thomas Y. Crowell, 1979. (H).

Paulin, Nadine L. *Home Aids for Recovery from Environmental Ill-*

ness: For the Patient; For the Family; For Friends. Potter Valley, California: Woods-Edge Press, n.d. (P)

Three pamphlets of practical tips.

Pfeiffer, Guy O., M.D., and Casimir M. Nikel. *The Household Environment and Chronic Illness-Guidelines for Constructing and Maintaining a Less-Polluted Residence.* Springfield, Illinois: Charles C. Thomas, 1980. (H)

A collection of informative and helpful articles aimed at pinpointing possibly harmful substances in the home, along with ways to correct the problems whether you are constructing your own home or buying a new or used home.

Philpott, William, M.D., and Dwight K. Kalita. Ph.D. *Brain Allergies.* New Canaan, Connecticut: Keats Publishing, Inc., 1980. (H)

A study of the connection between nutrition and mental illness.

————. *Victory Over Diabetes.* New Canaan, Connecticut: Keats Publishing, Inc., 1980. (H)

A bio-ecologic approach to the nature and treatment of diabetes based on the enhancement of and defense by the body's own resources.

Randolph, Theron G., M.D. *Human Ecology and Susceptibility to the Chemical Environment.* Springfield, Illinois: Charles C. Thomas, 1962. (H)

The classic introduction to environmental illness by the "Father of Clinical Ecology."

Randolph, Theron G., M.D. and Ralph W. Moss, Ph.D. *An Alternative Approach to Allergies.* New York: Lippincott & Crowell, 1980. (H)

An excellent exploration of the field of clinical ecology, with an emphasis on the philosophy of environmental medicine.

Rapp, Doris, J., M.D. *Allergies and the Hyperactive Child.* New York: Cornerstone Library, 1979. (P)

A pediatrician's look at how allergies relate to hyperactivity. A blending of clinical ecology with traditional allergy treatment. Even though ostensibly aimed at hyperactivity, it is a fairly generalized approach.

————. *Allergies and Your Family.* New York: Sterling Publishing Co., 1980. (P)

A pediatric allergist's look at allergies in easy-to-read question-and-answer style. A blending of clinical ecology with traditional allergy treatment.

————. *The Impossible Child*: Buffalo, New York: Practical Allergy Research Foundation, 1986. (P)

A practical, basic guide for recognizing and helping the hyperactive child at home and in the classroom. Written by a pediatric allergist for parents and teachers. Send $8.95 to the foundation, Box 60, Buffalo, NY 14223-0060.

Rinkel, Herbert J., M.D., Theron G. Randolph, M.D., and Michael Zeller, M.D. *Food Allergy.* Springfield, Illinois: Charles C. Thomas, 1951. (H)

An overview of food allergy by three pioneers in the field of clinical ecology. Its concise and clear approach makes it excellent reading for the well-read lay reader or professional.

Rowe, Albert H., M.D., and Albert Rowe, Jr., M.D. *Food Allergy-Its Manifestations and Control and the Elimination Diets.* Springfield, Illinois: Charles C. Thomas, 1972. (H)
> A clinical compendium of material on food and chemical allergies, appropriate for the medical profession and the well-read lay reader.

Saifer, Phyllis, M.D., M.P.H., and Merla Zellerback. *Detox.* Los Angeles: Jeremy P. Tarcher, Inc., 1984. ()

Sheinkin, David, M.D., Michael Schachter, M.D., and Richard Hutton, *Food, Mind & Mood* (original H Title: *The Food Connection*). New York: Warner Books, 1979. (P)
> An exploration of food allergy by two traditionally trained psychiatrists who found themselves drawn, through their patients' illnesses, to clinical ecology's approach to illness. A particular strength of this book is its nonjudgmental description, along with objective pros and cons, of most of the tests used by clinical ecologists.

Small, Bruce, and Barbara Small. *Sunnyhill.* Ontario: Small and Associates, 1980. (H)
> The personal story of a family's discovery of and fight against ecologic illness, culminating in their construction of an ecologically-sound home, which was designed to be a refuge for themselves and for other ecologically-ill people.

Taube, E. Louis, M.D. *Food Allergy and the Allergic Patient.* Springfield, Illinois: Charles C. Thomas, 1973. (P)
> A short, concise overview of the clinical ecologist's approach to treating food allergy, appropriate for the food-allergy patient who is just starting out.

Travis, Nick, and Ruth Holladay. *The Body Wrecker.* Amarillo, Texas: Don Quixote Publishing Co., 1981. (P)
> A two-part book: The first part is the story of a young man's near destruction by ecologic illness. The second part is an overview of clinical ecology, appropriate for, and aimed at, the lay reader.

U.S. Agriculture Handbook No. 456. *Nutritive Value of American Foods in Common Units.* Washington, D.C. 20204: Superintendent of Documents, Government Printing Office, 1975.

Appendix A: Formaldehyde Fact Sheet

Formaldehyde is the first member of the aldehyde group R-C-H, where R = H. Other common names include formalin and methanal. It is obtainable in gaseous or liquid form.

Uses of Formaldehyde

Formaldehyde has an unusual number of uses. It is widely used in the cosmetic industry and in the manufacture of a variety of household products. It is used in heavy manufacturing and chemical industries as well. Uses include the following:

- As intermediates in the synthesis of alcohols, acids, and other chemicals.
- As a tanning agent.
- In the formulation of slow-release nitrogen fertilizers, and in destroying microorganisms responsible for plant disease.
- As an additional agent to make concrete, plaster, and related products impermeable to liquids.
- As an antiperspirant, and as an antiseptic in dentifrices, mouthwashes, and germicidal and detergent soaps. It is also used in hair setting and in shampoos.
- As an air deodorant in public places and in industrial environments.
- To destroy bacteria, fungi, molds, and yeasts. It is used to disinfect equipment in the fermentation industries and in the manufacture of antibiotics. It is used to disinfect sickrooms and surgical instruments.
- As synthesis of dyes, stripping agents, and various specialty chemicals in the dye industry. It also improves the color stability of dyed fabrics.
- In combination with alcohol, glycerol, and phenol in embalming fluids. It is also used to preserve products such as waxes, polishes, adhesives, fats, oils, and anatomical specimens.
- As synthesis of explosives.
- In conjunction with other chemicals in preparing fireproofing compositions to apply to fabrics.

■ In insecticidal solutions for killing flies, mosquitoes, and moths. It is also used as a rodent poison.

■ In the synthesis of vitamin A and in improving the activity of vitamin E preparations.

■ To improve the wet strength and water resistance of paper products.

■ As a preservative and accelerator for photographic developing solutions.

■ To make natural and synthetic fibers crease-resistant, wrinkle-resistant, crush-proof, water-repellant, dye-fast, flame-resistant, water-resistant, shrink-proof, moth-proof (wool), and more elastic (wool).

■ In making synthetic resins, wood veneer (for wall paper), and to effect artificial aging, and reduction of shrinkage in wood preservation.

■ As one of the component parts of wallboard used in construction of houses and apartments.

■ As resin in nail polish and undercoating of nail polish.

Air Pollution

Formaldehyde usually accounts for about 50 percent of the estimated total aldehydes in polluted air. The major sources of aldehyde pollution are in the incomplete combustion of hydrocarbons in gasoline and diesel engines, burning of fuels, and incineration of waste. Formaldehyde is believed to be the principal agent responsible for the burning of the eyes in smog. Aldehydes can also react further to form products such as additional ozone.

Nationwide spot-checks show the following ambient air sources of aldehydes:

formaldehyde producing plants	2,580 ppm
gasoline autos	50–100 malfunctioning
combustion of coal	.06–.25
fuel oil combustion	3–52
natural gas combustion	5–15
incinerator	49
small domestic incinerators	1–67
backyard incinerators	760
petroleum refineries	3–130

drying ovens	52
small batch auto incinerators	16
aircraft	5 idling, 1 takeoff
baking of lithographic coatings	12–186

Appendix B: Alcohol Fact Sheet

This is the class name for a group of chemicals recognized as having a certain definite chemical make-up, containing one or more carbinol groups. This is written C-O-H. H is a hydrogen atom attached to an oxygen atom, which is also attached to a carbon atom. This carbon atom has at least three other attachments.

Alcohol: Kinds and Uses

The above formulas result in a variety of alcohols. They include the following:

1 **Ethyl Alcohol** is formed by the action of yeast on sugar (molasses) or from starch (potatoes and corn). Ethyl alcohol

- Will dissolve many organic substances, such as shellac and oil.
- Is used as body rubbing alcohol.
- Is used in making ether and in sterilizing surgical instruments.
- Is an ingredient in tinctures and many toilet and drug preparations.
- Is used in making rubber.

2 **Amyl Alcohol** is made from ethyl alcohol. It is used as a solvent.

3 **Methyl Alcohol** is a fatal poison, prepared by the destructive distillation of wood. It is used in preparing formaldehyde and as a solvent for varnishes and lacquers.

4 **Isopropyl Alcohol** is used in manufacture of antifreeze, rubbing alcohol, and solvents.

5 **Butyl Alcohol** is made from grain and potatoes. It is used in making synthetic rubber and insulation.

6 **Ethylene Glycol** is prepared by the action of sulphuric acid and ethyl alcohol and is used in the production of antifreeze.

7 **Glycerol** is composed of carbon, hydrogen, and oxygen, and is obtained from fats as a by-product in the manufacture of soaps and fatty acids. Glycerol is

- Used for sweetening and preserving food.

■ Used in the manufacture of cosmetics, perfumes, inks, and certain glues and cements.

■ Used in medicine in suppositories and skin emollients.

8 Menthol is composed of carbon, hydrogen, and the hydroxyl (OH) group. It is used in perfumes, confections, and liqueurs. Menthol is also used in medicine for colds and nasal disorders because of its cooling effect on mucous membranes.

Products of Alcohol:

Alcohol is one of the most widely used chemical compounds. The following lists provide only suggestions of the many uses. Those who are sensitive to alcohol should read the labels of all products that the following list includes or suggests.

acetic acid	flavoring extract	preservatives
anesthetics	hand lotions	printers's ink
celluloid	nylon textiles	rayon textiles
cleaning fluid	paint and varnish	rubber overshoes
drugs	perfumes	rubber tires
dyes	photographic film	soaps
explosives	plastics	synthetic chemicals

Appendix C: Phenol Fact Sheet

Phenol is any of a family of organic compounds characterized by attachment of at least one hydroxyl group to a carbon atom forming part of the benzene ring.

Phenol is also called carbolic acid or hydroxybenzene. In 1834, a German, named Runge, isolated carbolic acid from coal tar. In 1843, another German, Gerhardt, prepared the same substance by a different method and called it "phenol." In 1845, an English surgeon, Joseph Lister began to use a dilute solution of phenol to treat wounds, establishing its usage as an antiseptic.

Uses:

Like alcohol and formaldehyde, phenol is very widely used in industry. Those who are sensitive to this chemical are advised to read carefully the labels of the many products that the following list of substances and uses suggest.

- Phenol is the starting point for the production of epoxy and phenolic resins, aspirin, and other drugs.
- Used in the manufacture of picric acid explosives.
- A constituent of herbicides and pesticides.
- Used in making molded articles, such as telephone parts, thermal insulation panels and laminated boards, children's toys, refrigerator storage dishes, etc.
- Used in the manufacture of nylon.
- Used in the manufacture of synthetic detergents.
- Used in the manufacture of polyurathene.
- Used in the manufacture of perfume.
- Used in the manufacture of gasoline additives.
- Used in the manufacture of dyes.
- Used in the manufacture of photography solutions.
- A preservative in medications; a preservative for antigen serum in allergy shots.

There are naturally occurring phenols, such as the toxic agent in poison ivy and poison oak. Thyme oil, from thyme, is used as an intermediate solution in the production of menthol. Phenol may occur in spring water as a result of humus in or around the spring or from natural coal in the ground around the spring.

Appendix D: Tri Alkali Salts Fact Sheet

One of the most effective procedures to counteract food or chemical reaction is the use of Tri Alkali Salts. *This procedure should only be used with the prescription of your doctor.* If you believe it would be beneficial for you, consult your doctor and follow his prescription. This section is offered only as a reference for your information. On the advice of your physician, you may want to annotate this material to suit your needs. You may wish to put your name and date with your notes, in case you share this textbook with someone else.

Composition of Tri Alkali Salts

3 parts sodium bicarbonate
2 parts potassium bicarbonate
1 part calcium carbonate.

Purpose

To neutralize withdrawal symptoms and counteract acidosis resulting from chemical or food reactions, and to clean out the gastrointestinal tract. These reactions may come from unexpected exposure on food testing done under a physician's supervision.

Dosage

Adults: One teaspoonful in a quarter glass of water, followed by two glasses of water.
Children: half the amount of adult dose for half body weight.

When to Use

During withdrawal and to counteract food or chemical reaction. Allergic reactions interfere with natural buffering system, producing intracellular edema and acidosis.

Tri Salts given orally or rectally will neutralize this acidosis, help reduce the edema, and act as a saline laxative. The earlier the Tri Salts are administered during the first twenty-four hours after the onset of an acute reaction, the more effective they will be.

When Not To Use

Acute reactions for as long as twenty-four hours, status asthmaticus, symptoms lasting more than twenty-four hours, such as continued headache, advanced mental reactions, persistent depression, and Ménière's syndrome are made worse by alkali salts. They increase the edema, resulting in occluded airways or increased brain swelling. CAUTION: *Patients with heart conditions and kidney difficulties may never use salts unless prescribed by the doctor.*

Appendix E: Use of Milk of Magnesia

Purpose

To help with emptying of gastrointestinal tract during withdrawal.

Average Dosage

Four tablespoons, followed by two glasses of water. (Some patients may need more, some patients less.)

When to Use

During withdrawal and when reacting to ingested food.

Miscellaneous Uses

May be applied to skin to soothe rashes when other medication cannot be used. May be applied to lips in case of chapping or dry lips.

Appendix F: HEAL Membership Application

We reproduce a membership application form for the Human Ecology Action League, the value of which we hope has been made clear in the text. You may copy it or sacrifice the page it's on, but you will benefit from using it.

Mail to: HEAL Inc., 2421 West Pratt, Suite 1112, Chicago IL 60645

Human Ecology Action League Membership Application

First Name_____Initial_____Last Name_____

Address_____

City_____State_____Zip_____

Member/Subscriber Dues	Additional Contributions

Member/Subscriber Dues

☐ U.S. $20
☐ Canada/Mexico $25
☐ Other Countries ... $28

Additional Contributions

☐ Friend ..... $10   ☐ Patron $50
☐ Contributor $25   ☐ Sponsor ... $100
☐ Benefactor ... $100 +

Foreign: Please send
U.S. Funds

Above listed in *The Human Ecologist*. Check here *only* if anonymity preferred. ☐

Other Information

Do you want your name to be given to a HEAL Chapter existing or beginning in your area? ☐ Yes ☐ No

Do you want your name given to a HEAL member seeking to contact others in your area? ☐ Yes ☐ No

Note: ☐ New ☐ Renewal ☐ Address Change

HEAL is a non-profit organization and member/subscriber dues and contributions are tax deductible.